The APIC/JCR

Infection Prevention and Control Workbook

Second Edition

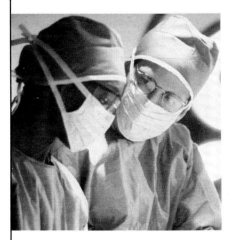
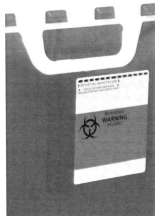
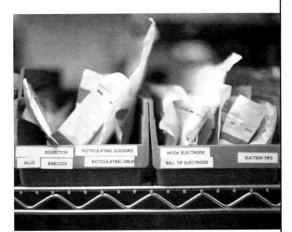
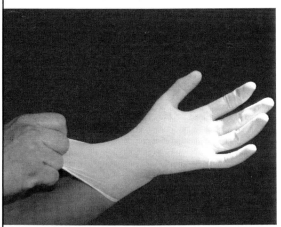
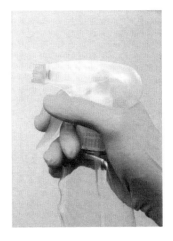
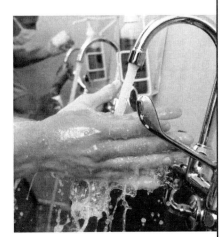

Joint Commission Resources

 APIC

EDITED BY

Kathleen Meehan Arias,
M.S., C.I.C.

Barbara Moore Soule,
R.N., M.P.A., C.I.C.

Executive Editor: Kristine M. Miller, M.F.A.
Project Manager: Bridget Chambers
Managers, Publications: Victoria Gaudette, Paul Reis, Diane Bell
Associate Director, Production: Johanna Harris
Executive Director: Catherine Chopp Hinckley, Ph.D.

APIC Reviewers:
Amy M. Richmond, R.N., B.S.N., M.H.S., C.I.C., Infection Preventionist, Barnes-Jewish Hospital, St. Louis, Missouri

APIC Coordinator:
Nick Hill, Associate Director, Product Development

Joint Commission Reviewers:
Pat Adamski, R.N., M.S., M.B.A., Director, Standards Interpretation Group and The Office of Quality Monitoring, Division of Accreditation and Certification Operations
Carol Mooney, R.N., M.S.N., Senior Associate Director, Standards Interpretation Group, Accreditation and Certification Operations
Laurel Shine, R.N., M.S., C.P.H.Q., Associate Director, Standards Interpretation Group
Louise Kuhny, R.N., M.P.H., M.B.A., C.I.C., Senior Associate Director, Standards Interpretation Group
Cynthia Leslie, A.P.R.N., M.S.N., B.C., Associate Director, Standards Interpretation Group
Jerry Gervais, C.H.F.M, C.H.S.P, Associate Director/Engineer, Standards Interpretation Group
John D. Maurer, C.H.F.M, C.H.S.P, Associate Director/Engineer, Standards Interpretation Group

Joint Commission Resources Reviewer:
Deborah M. Nadzam, Ph.D., F.A.A.N., Practice Leader, Patient Safety Services

Joint Commission Resources Mission
The mission of Joint Commission Resources is to continuously improve the safety and quality of care in the United States and in the international community through the provision of education and consultation services and international accreditation.

Joint Commission Resources educational programs and publications support, but are separate from, the accreditation activities of The Joint Commission. Attendees at Joint Commission Resources educational programs and purchasers of Joint Commission Resources publications receive no special consideration or treatment in, or confidential information about, the accreditation process.

The inclusion of an organization name, a product, or a service in a Joint Commission publication should not be construed as an endorsement of such organization, product, or service, nor is failure to include an organization name, a product, or a service to be construed as disapproval.

This publication is designed to provide accurate and authoritative information regarding the subject matter covered. Every attempt has been made to ensure accuracy at the time of publication; however, please note that laws, regulations, and standards are subject to change. Please also note that some of the examples in this publication are specific to the laws and regulations of the locality of the facility. The information and examples in this publication are provided with the understanding that the publisher is not engaged in providing medical, legal, or other professional advice. If any such assistance is desired, the services of a competent professional person should be sought.

ISBN: 978-1-59940-313-7

Library of Congress Control Number: 2009943575

For more information about Joint Commission Resources, please visit http://www.jcrinc.com.

Contents

Contributors

Kathleen Meehan Arias, M.S., C.I.C.
Arias Infection Control Consulting, LLC
Crownsville, Maryland

Ruth M. Carrico, Ph.D., R.N., C.I.C.
Assistant Professor
School of Public Health and Information Sciences
University of Louisville
Louisville, Kentucky

Loretta Litz Fauerbach, M.S., C.I.C.
Director, Infection Prevention and Control
Shands Hospital at the University of Florida/Shands
    HealthCare
Gainesville, Florida

Candace Friedman, M.P.H., C.I.C.
Director, Infection Control and Epidemiology
University of Michigan Health System
Ann Arbor, Michigan

Louise Kuhny, R.N., M.P.H., M.B.A., C.I.C.
Senior Associate Director
Standards Interpretation Group
The Joint Commission
Oakbrook Terrace, Illinois

Tammy S. Lundstrom, M.D., J.D.
Chief Medical Officer
Providence Hospital
Southfield, Michigan

Russell N. Olmsted, M.P.H., C.I.C.
Epidemiologist, Infection Prevention and Control Services
Saint Joseph Mercy Health System
Ann Arbor, Michigan

Shannon Oriola, R.N., C.I.C., C.O.H.N.
Department Lead, Infection Prevention and Clinical
    Epidemiology
Sharp Metropolitan Medical Campus
San Diego, California

Terri Rebmann, Ph.D., R.N., C.I.C.
Associate Director for Curricular Affairs
Assistant Professor, Institute for Biosecurity
Saint Louis University, School of Public Health
St. Louis, Missouri

Sue Sebazco, R.N., B.S., C.I.C.
Infection Prevention/Employee Health Director
Texas Health Arlington Memorial Hospital
Arlington, Texas

Susan M. Slavish, B.S.N., M.P.H., C.I.C.
Consultant, Joint Commission Resources
Oak Brook, Illinois

Barbara Moore Soule, R.N., M.P.A., C.I.C.
Practice Leader, Infection Prevention Services
Joint Commission Resources and Joint Commission
    International
Oak Brook, Illinois

Foreword

Today more than ever, infection prevention and control is one of the most pressing patient safety issues facing health care organizations. Health care–associated infections (HAIs) can exact a heavy price, both in resources and in human lives. Emerging pathogens such as the newer, more toxic strains of *Clostridium difficile* require intense efforts to prevent their spread, and infectious diseases such as the novel influenza A (H1N1) bring the specter of pandemic closer to reality and challenge organizations' abilities to cope. Moreover, growing media attention and consumer concern about the significant number of deaths and other adverse outcomes caused by HAIs intensify the urgency for health care organizations to ensure that they have adequate resources allocated to prevent and control infections. From the smallest facility to the most complex health care system, an organization-appropriate infection prevention and control program must be part of an organization's overall strategy and long-term planning.

This freshly updated edition of *The APIC/JCR Infection Prevention and Control Workbook,* second edition, addresses these and many other issues. It reflects the revised Joint Commission "Infection Prevention and Control" (IC) standards, which were thoroughly reorganized and clarified to help organizations better manage their infection prevention and control programs, as well as the Joint Commission's significantly expanded National Patient Safety Goals. The book also incorporates the most up-to-date information in the continually evolving science and practice of infection prevention and control. And it highlights the increased emphasis on performance improvement and patient safety in the infection prevention arena.

The APIC/JCR Infection Prevention and Control Workbook, second edition, is the product of a fruitful collaboration between the Association for Professionals in Infection Control and Epidemiology (APIC) and Joint Commission Resources (JCR), the publishing affiliate of The Joint Commission. In this book, leading experts in infection prevention and control from APIC and JCR offer practical guidance to help health care organizations improve their infection prevention and control systems and processes. The authors' firsthand experiences provide invaluable perspective and insight into current issues and challenges in infection prevention. The authors provide key tips and strategies and offer a wealth of successful examples from health care organizations of all types.

This workbook is intended to be a hands-on tool that can be used in conjunction with your organization's ongoing efforts to assess, improve, and fine-tune its infection prevention and control program and to achieve compliance with the Joint Commission IC standards. It can help you gauge your own successes to date and implement improvements, plus it provides important education and information to infection preventionists new to the field.

With ongoing risks for HAIs, emerging infectious diseases, and antimicrobial-resistant pathogens and the ongoing possibility of natural disasters and bioterrorism, health care organizations must continually make the changes and improvements to minimize impact on patient safety. We believe this workbook will help you improve the quality and safety of the care you provide to your patients.

Karen H. Timmons
President and CEO, *Joint Commission Resources*

Kathy L. Warye
CEO, *Association for Professionals in
Infection Control and Epidemiology*

ACKNOWLEDGMENTS

A work of this scope requires a concerted team effort. This book, which we hope you find to be as useful as it is practical, could not have been created without such a team. We are deeply indebted to our content editors, Kathleen Meehan Arias, M.S., C.I.C., and Barbara Moore Soule, R.N., M.P.A., C.I.C., whose intense labors and masterful professional expertise ensured the high quality of this product; our chapter contributors, whose expert insight has added depth and relevancy to the topics under discussion (see page vii for a complete listing of names); and the many organizations which contributed the outstanding tools and examples that enrich this book.

We express our profound gratitude to our writer, Kathleen B. Vega, for her consummate journalistic expertise, careful attention to detail, and outstanding professionalism.

We are grateful to our APIC coordinator and our APIC, Joint Commission Resources, and Joint Commission reviewers (see page ii) for their thorough and timely input.

Chapter 1

Setting the Stage: An Introduction

Barbara Moore Soule, R.N., M.P.A., C.I.C.; and Louise Kuhny, R.N., M.P.H., M.B.A., C.I.C.

Millions of people each year acquire infections while receiving treatment in health care organizations, and some of these people never recover. According to the Centers for Disease Control and Prevention (CDC), 1.7 million infections annually are related to health care settings, and these infections lead to 99,000 deaths each year.[1]

Infections can be acquired in virtually all health care settings, and no organization is immune. Although it is true that some patients and residents who acquire infections in health care organizations are frail, elderly, or immunocompromised, healthy people also enter health care organizations for elective procedures or rehabilitation, fully expecting to return home in good health, and instead acquire infections that sometimes result in death.

Until recently, many people in health care believed that health care–associated infections (HAIs) are a regrettable but inevitable consequence of complex care delivered to increasingly sick patients. In other words, they believed that HAIs are collateral damage in the challenging pursuit of medicine. However, with the right interventions, education, and organizational commitment, the transmission of HAIs, along with other infections, can be reduced.

The fact is that despite the number of infections and the potentially severe consequences associated with infections, organizations can effect change in this area. Consequently, the surveillance, prevention, and control of infections represents one of the most significant patient safety initiatives in a health care organization and should be a top priority for all organizations.

CREATING A COMPREHENSIVE INFECTION PREVENTION AND CONTROL PROGRAM

To help reduce the impact of infections and the likelihood of transmission, health care organizations need to create a systematic and proactive infection prevention and control (IPC) program. This program should be based on the specific infection risks an organization faces, the services it provides, and the populations it serves. Such a program should stress communication and collaboration and be based on accepted best practices regarding infection prevention and control.

A strong IPC program has the input, involvement, and endorsement of leadership as well as frontline staff. In fact, everyone involved in the daily operations of an organization—including clinical staff, administrative staff, environmental services staff, and so on—should play a role in developing, implementing, and sustaining the IPC program.

Because the infection risks, services provided, and populations served by an organization can change, regular evaluation of the IPC program is important. As part of evaluation efforts, organizations must use evaluation data to modify the IPC program to ensure that the most appropriate infection prevention and control strategies are in place.

WHAT THE JOINT COMMISSION REQUIRES REGARDING INFECTION PREVENTION AND CONTROL

The Joint Commission addresses the topic of infection prevention and control through both its standards and its National Patient Safety Goals. Fundamentally, the "Infection Prevention and Control" (IC) standards are designed to assist a health care organization, both large or small, in developing and maintaining an effective IPC program that covers a wide range of infection-related situations. The standards address activities of planning, implementation, and evaluation and outline the role of the infection preventionist, organization leadership, and frontline staff. Specifically, the standards address the following issues:

- Allocating resources to an IPC program
- Ensuring that staff are competent and have clinical IPC knowledge
- Ensuring leadership buy-in and support of the IPC program
- Creating an IPC plan based on risk assessment and prioritization
- Managing an infection control emergency or outbreak
- Using evidence-based practices regarding infection prevention and control
- Ensuring effective communication—both internally and externally—about infection prevention and control issues
- Managing infection risks in the environment of care
- Ensuring occupational health through proactive screenings, vaccinations, and immunizations
- Evaluating the IPC program

As previously mentioned, the Joint Commission also addresses infection prevention and control in its National Patient Safety Goals. The goals related to infection prevention and control require organizations to implement a comprehensive hand hygiene program, prevent HAIs related to multidrug-resistant organisms, prevent central line–associated bloodstream infections, and prevent surgical site infections.

The IC standards and National Patient Safety Goals work together to help an organization realize a comprehensive IPC program that is able to respond to the ever-changing infection risks present in a health care organization.

USING THE *APIC/JCR INFECTION PREVENTION AND CONTROL WORKBOOK*

To help organizations develop, implement, and evaluate an IPC program, the Association for Professionals in Infection

Control and Epidemiology (APIC) and Joint Commission Resources (JCR) have collaborated to produce *The APIC/JCR Infection Prevention and Control Workbook*, second edition, which addresses infection prevention issues in a variety of health care settings. Involving the input of experienced and knowledgeable infection preventionists, the purpose of this hands-on workbook is to take an organization through the most challenging infection prevention–related issues and explore the patient-centric concepts behind the Joint Commission's IC standards, other relevant standards, and the National Patient Safety Goals related to infection prevention and control. Each chapter in the workbook is written by an expert or experts in the field of infection prevention and control and discusses a different aspect of the standards and National Patient Safety Goals—providing compliance suggestions and offering figures, forms, tables, and tools to help organizations with compliance efforts. Many of the figures and tables from the text of the book, many are accessible via the "CD Tools" section on the enclosed CD.

By using this workbook, infection preventionists and others who work in the organization, such as organization leadership, occupational health professionals, environment of care staff, clinical staff, and other health care staff, can work together to develop a comprehensive IPC program and preserve the safety of patients and staff while reducing the introduction and transmission of infectious diseases within the organization.

REFERENCE

1. Centers for Disease Control and Prevention: *Estimates of Healthcare-Associated Infections.* http://www.cdc.gov/ncidod/dhqp/hai.html (accessed Jul. 7, 2009).

Chapter 2

The Infection Prevention and Control Program

Kathleen Meehan Arias, M.S., C.I.C.

Health care–associated infections (HAIs) cause considerable morbidity and mortality and are recognized as a patient safety problem.[1,2] Although it is not known what portion of HAIs are preventable,[3] it has long been recognized that an effective infection prevention and control (IPC) program reduces the risk of HAIs and improves health care outcomes.[4,5] For example, the Study on the Efficacy of Nosocomial Infection Control (SENIC) Project, conducted in the 1970s, demonstrated that hospitals that had intensive infection surveillance and control programs were able to reduce their infection rates by 32%.[4] In recent years, collaborative and individual facility performance improvement initiatives have demonstrated substantial reductions in HAI rates.[6,7] A growing body of evidence suggests that the portion of HAIs that are preventable may be greater than previously believed.

A contemporary IPC program should aim to reduce the occurrence of HAIs to the lowest possible levels. This chapter discusses how to allocate resources for an effective IPC program and reduce the occurrence of HAIs.

MANAGING AN EFFECTIVE INFECTION PREVENTION AND CONTROL PROGRAM

An effective IPC program has several important components. Whereas some of these components have remained constant throughout the years, others are evolving. For example, the essential components of the effective IPC programs in the SENIC Project included the following:

- Organized surveillance and control activities
- One infection preventionist for every 250 hospital beds
- A trained, effectual hospital epidemiologist
- A system for reporting infection rates to practicing surgeons[4]

Since the 1970s, infection surveillance, prevention, and control programs have extended beyond the acute care hospital to include a variety of health care settings, such as long term care, ambulatory care, same-day surgical centers, behavioral health care facilities, rehabilitation care facilities, and home care, to meet the needs of a changing health care delivery system.[8] In addition to expanded scope, the responsibilities of the IPC program have grown beyond infection prevention and control to include other issues, such as performance improvement, patient safety, occupational health, construction, emergency preparedness, and mandatory reporting.[9] It is now well accepted that the number of infection preventionists needed to staff an effective IPC program cannot be based on bed size alone[10] but should take into account the complexities of the organization and the scope of the program. (*See* page 11 for a further discussion of appropriate staffing for IPC programs.) Regardless of an organization's type or size, the infection surveillance, prevention, and control program must meet the organization's needs and comply with applicable standards, guidelines, regulations, and other requirements.

Successful implementation of IPC programs across the continuum of care depends on adequate numbers of trained personnel responsible for the daily management of the programs' activities. These activities include the following:

- Assessing, analyzing, and eliminating the risks of HAIs
- Conducting surveillance activities
- Monitoring trends in antimicrobial resistance
- Educating clinical staff about strategies to prevent infection
- Participating in performance improvement and patient safety activities
- Ensuring that evidence-based infection prevention practices are used

- Identifying and managing outbreaks
- Monitoring the effectiveness of the IPC program
- Communicating with staff and leadership

(*See* Sidebar 2-1, below, for a list of the essential components of an effective IPC program, regardless of setting.)

EXPLORING IC.01.01.01

The Joint Commission standards specifically state that an organization's leaders must assign one or more individuals to

---

Sidebar 2-1: The Components of an Effective Infection Prevention and Control (IPC) Program

- System for obtaining, managing, and reporting critical data and information
- Risk assessment for each care setting
- Written IPC plan based on risk assessment
- Organized surveillance program
- Use of surveillance findings in performance assessment and improvement activities
- Capacity to identify epidemiologically important organisms, outbreaks, and clusters of infectious disease
- Internal and external communication systems
- Written policies and procedures based on evidence-based practices
- Compliance with applicable regulations, standards, guidelines, and other requirements
- Integration with the employee health program
- Authority to implement infection prevention and control measures
- Education and training programs
- Trained personnel
- Nonpersonnel resources, such as computers, information technology, and laboratory support
- Integration with emergency preparedness systems in the organization and community
- Collaboration with the health department

Source: Adapted from Scheckler W.E., et al.: Requirements for infrastructure and essential activities of infection control and epidemiology in hospitals: A consensus panel report. *Am J Infect Control* 26:47–60, Feb. 1998; and Friedman C., et al.: Requirements for infrastructure and essential activities of infection control and epidemiology in out-of-hospital settings: A consensus panel report. *Am J Infect Control* 27:418–430, Oct. 1999.

---

be responsible for the IPC program and that leaders must allocate adequate resources for the program.

STANDARD IC.01.01.01

The [organization] identifies the individual(s) responsible for the infection prevention and control program.

The following sections discuss the Joint Commission's elements of performance (EPs) for Standard IC.01.01.01 and provide examples of effective strategies and interventions for incorporating these elements into an IPC program in a variety of health care settings. This chapter provides guidance for meeting this standard, Chapter 3 contains additional information about allocating resources.

IC.01.01.01, EP 1: The [organization] identifies the individual(s) with clinical authority over the infection prevention and control program.

To comply with this EP, organizations should consider the following activities:

- *Identify the individual(s).* An organization should assign responsibility for the supervision of the IPC program to one or more individuals, based on the organization's size, type, complexity, and populations served. The individual(s) assigned should have knowledge of the clinical principles and practices used to prevent and control the transmission of infection, as discussed in the section "IC.01.01.01, EP 3."
- *Designate authority for action.* The person(s) responsible for supervising the IPC program should have the authority to take action quickly when steps that are needed to prevent or control the spread of infectious agents are identified. For example, if the infection preventionist in a long term care facility learns that a resident has respiratory symptoms and many acid-fast bacilli in his sputum, the infection preventionist should have the authority to immediately implement airborne precautions or, if the long term care facility does not have that capability, to begin the process of transferring the resident to another facility that has the capacity to isolate airborne diseases.

Although not specifically required in the current Joint Commission standards, most organizations have a written statement that authorizes specified personnel, such as the infection preventionist and/or health care epidemiologist and/or that person's designee, to institute appropriate control measures when there is deemed to be infection danger to patients and health care workers. Such control measures may include the following:

— Instituting isolation precautions for a patient or resident
— Ordering cultures or other laboratory tests
— Restricting visitors
— Temporarily closing a unit or ward to further admissions in case of a suspected or actual outbreak
— Restricting movement of patients or residents from one area to another

Some states require an organization to have an authority statement for the infection preventionist and/or for a physician member of the Infection Prevention and Control Committee. An example of an authority statement follows in the box below.

SAMPLE AUTHORITY STATEMENT

The Infection Preventionist and the Hospital Epidemiologist, through the authority of the Infection Prevention and Control Committee, have the authority to institute appropriate control measures when danger to a patient or personnel is reasonably felt to be present. Examples of such control measures include:

1. Institution of appropriate isolation precautions, in accordance with the Isolation Policies and Procedures outlined in the *Infection Prevention and Control Manual*;
2. Initiation of culture and sensitivity testing in the face of obvious indication;
3. Provision of in-service education for personnel on such topics as the proper use of aseptic technique and strategies for preventing the transmission of infectious agents;
4. Initiation of studies needed to identify the source, reservoir and/or mode of transmission of an outbreak of health care–associated infections; and
5. Initiation of other control measures as deemed necessary based on surveillance findings and reports of infections and infection potential among patients and personnel.

Source: Arias Infection Control Consulting, LLC. Used with permission.

• *Create a job description.* The organization should provide an appropriate job description for all infection preventionist and health care epidemiologist positions, as applicable. The job description should include the position title, reporting structure, job summary, qualifications, and duties and responsibilities. (An example of a job description for an infection preventionist can found in Figure 2-1 on page 6 and in the "CD tools" section for this chapter.)

IC.01.01.01, EP 2: When the individual(s) with clinical authority over the infection prevention and control program does not have expertise in infection prevention and control, he or she consults with someone who has such expertise in order to make knowledgeable decisions. (*See also* IC.01.02.01, EP 1.)

If the individual(s) assigned to manage the IPC program does not have expertise in infection prevention and control, the organization's leadership is responsible for identifying an experienced infection preventionist and/or hospital epidemiologist who can assist in making knowledgeable decisions relating to infection prevention and control. These experienced personnel may be employees of the organization, contractual agents, or outside consultants. For example, the leaders of a long term care facility may arrange for an infection preventionist from a local hospital or the epidemiologist from an academic medical center to provide consultation services, as needed, to assist the on-site person assigned responsibility for managing the facility's IPC program.

IC.01.01.01, EP 3: The organization assigns responsibility for the daily management of infection prevention and control activities. (*See also* HR.01.02.01, EP 1, and LD.02.01.01, EP 3.) *Note:* Number and skill mix of the individual(s) assigned should be determined by the goals and objectives of the infection prevention and control program.

When considering how to comply with IC.01.01.01, EP 3, organizations should keep in mind the following points:

■ *Ensure leadership involvement.* The organization's leaders must be directly involved in determining the personnel and nonpersonnel resources needed for the IPC program. (*See* Chapter 3.) Regardless of the health care setting, the responsibility for the daily management of the IPC program should be clearly assigned to at least one person who is knowledgeable about infectious

Figure 2-1. Job Description for an Infection Preventionist

Job Title:	Infection Preventionist
Date created: Date revised:	
FLSA Status:	

Job Summary

Coordinates comprehensive organizationwide infection prevention and control program in accordance with current requirements of regulatory, government, and accrediting/licensing agencies and organizational policies and procedures. Duties include surveillance for health care–associated infections (HAIs); collection, analysis, and interpretation of surveillance data; outbreak investigation; and program evaluation. Responsible for the day-to-day administration and development of the infection prevention and control program.

Reporting Structure

Reports to the Vice President, Quality Improvement.

Major Duties

1. Develops and maintains an infection surveillance, prevention, and control program based on the organization's risk assessment and other needs and in accordance with state, federal, and other reporting requirements
2. Collects, manages, and analyzes surveillance data using standardized methodology and defined criteria for an HAI
3. Organizes and maintains surveillance data and records
4. Reports surveillance data, findings, and analyses to the appropriate committees, patient care units, personnel, and external agencies
5. Monitors patients for the occurrence of communicable diseases, HAIs, and resistant and epidemiologically important organisms
6. Monitors infectious diseases and epidemiologically significant organisms occurring in the community via laboratory reports and public health reports
7. Identifies and evaluates clusters of infections and potential outbreaks
8. Institutes an outbreak investigation and control measures, as needed
9. Recommends isolation precautions according to organization's policies and procedures
10. Develops infection prevention and control policies and protocols in accordance with requirements of regulatory, government, and accrediting/licensing agencies and recommendations of relevant professional organizations
11. Updates policies and protocols, as needed, to maintain compliance with regulations, standards, and evidence-based guidelines
12. Assists the organization to evaluate and maintain readiness for state and accrediting agency surveys
13. Monitors and evaluates the efficacy of infection prevention and control strategies
14. Collaborates with all departments of the facility to design and implement strategies to prevent HAIs and transmission of multidrug-resistant organisms and other epidemiologically important organisms
15. Investigates exposures to communicable disease and initiates appropriate measures to prevent the transmission of disease
16. Maintains confidentiality of patients, personnel, and related information
17. Provides consultation services relating to infection prevention and control to the various departments in the organization
18. Evaluates products, devices, and equipment as relating to infection prevention and control

(continued)

Figure 2-1. Job Description for an Infection Preventionist (continued)

19. Actively participates in performance improvement activities
20. Maintains departmental records to be in compliance with regulatory and accrediting agencies
21. Provides written and verbal reports to administration and relevant committees, departments, personnel, and external agencies
22. Communicates with local and state health departments
23. Participates in orientation programs and required annual education programs
24. Conducts in-service education on hand hygiene, aseptic technique, infection prevention and control strategies, antiseptics and disinfectants, specific infectious diseases, and other related health care issues
25. Develops or obtains educational materials and programs, as needed, for personnel, patients, and visitors
26. Collaborates with employee health personnel on matters such as exposure management and immunization
27. Works with facilities management and other personnel to evaluate infection risks associated with renovation and construction projects and to identify control measures
28. Is an active member of the following committees: Infection Prevention and Control, Patient Care Council, Quality and Performance Improvement, and Product Standardization

Qualifications
- ___ years' experience in clinical/patient care services or relevant health care position
- Minimum of B.S. Degree in Nursing, Microbiology, Public Health, Medical Technology, or related field required. Related license or certification.
- CIC certification preferred. Ability to take certification examination after 3 years or less of employment required.

Knowledge/skills/abilities
- Familiarity with relevant state, federal, and accrediting agency requirements
- Knowledge and experience in areas of patient care practices, microbiology, asepsis, disinfection and sterilization, adult education, infectious diseases, epidemiology, statistics, communication, and program administration
- Self-motivated, organized, and detail oriented
- Ability to collect, analyze, and report data
- Computer literacy, including Microsoft Office (Word, Excel, Access, and PowerPoint) and ability to obtain, enter, and manage data using a computer
- Excellent oral and written communication skills
- Ability to facilitate performance improvement initiatives
- Able to organize and manage time and multiple tasks
- Participates in ongoing self-education and professional development
- Is an active member of relevant professional organization(s)
- Adheres to the principles and to the mission of the organization
- Ability to manage infection prevention and control department staff (when applicable)

The above statements are intended to describe the general duties and level of work performed by those persons assigned to this position. These statements are not designed to contain or be interpreted as a comprehensive inventory of all duties, responsibilities, and qualifications required of employees assigned to the job. Management retains the discretion to add to or change the duties of the position at any time.

This figure shows a comprehensive job description for an infection preventionist that can be adapted to an organization's specific needs. FLSA, Fair Labor Standards Act; CIC, Certified in Infection Control.

Source: Arias Infection Control Consulting, LLC. Used with permission.

diseases, infection risks, the principles of infection prevention and control, and data collection, analysis, and presentation.[11–13]

■ *Verify core competencies.* Infection preventionists come from different professional backgrounds, such as nursing, medical technology, microbiology, medicine, and other health care fields, and have varying academic preparation and degrees. Regardless of background or training, an infection preventionist should strive to attain certain competencies to manage an effective infection surveillance, prevention, and control program. The person(s) assigned to the program should demonstrate basic knowledge relating to the following areas:

Epidemiology, including outbreak management; infectious diseases; microbiology; patient care practices; asepsis; disinfection/sterilization; occupational health; facility planning and construction; emergency preparedness; learning/education principles; communication; product evaluation; information technology; program administration; legislative issues/policy making; and research.[13]

Professional and practice standards for an infection preventionist have been developed by a task force appointed by the boards of directors of the Association for Professionals in Infection Control and Epidemiology (APIC), the Community and Hospital Infection Control Association of Canada (CHICA–Canada), and the Certification Board of Infection Control and Epidemiology (CBIC).[13] A list of core competencies, based on the APIC/CHICA–Canada standards[13] and recommendations of two consensus panels convened by the Society for Healthcare Epidemiology of America (SHEA),[11,12] is included in Sidebar 2-2 on page 00. (Refer to the cited references for additional information.)

TIP: *Regardless of background or training, an infection preventionist should strive to attain certain competencies to manage an effective infection surveillance, prevention, and control program.*

To help ensure that a new infection preventionist is competent to manage its IPC program, an organization should provide an orientation program to present an overview of the responsibilities of the position and the core competencies expected. (Figure 2-2 on page 9 shows a checklist organizations can use

---

Sidebar 2-2: Core Competencies for the Infection Preventionist

- Meets recommended qualifications for the profession
  ○ Is an experienced health care professional with health sciences background
  ○ Has working knowledge of patient care practices, microbiology, asepsis, disinfection and sterilization practices, adult education principles, infectious diseases, communication methods, program administration, epidemiology and disease transmission, surveillance techniques, statistical measures used in infection prevention and control, occupational health issues, performance measurement and improvement principles, and standards, regulations, and other requirements affecting infection prevention and control (IPC) programs
- Participates in professional development
  ○ Remains current in infection prevention and control practices (for example, by attending formal educational programs and meetings, networking with other infection preventionists, reading infection prevention and control and infectious disease literature, and using technology such as the Internet and e-mail alerts to obtain the latest information)
  ○ Attends a basic training course in infection prevention and control within the first six months of entering the profession
  ○ Strives to become certified in infection control by the Certification Board of Infection Control and Epidemiology[14]
  ○ Uses information technology for data collection, management, and reporting and for communication with others
  ○ Participates in related professional organizations
- Serves as a leader by collaborating with others and sharing information and expertise
- Makes decisions and performs duties in an ethical manner
- Holds self professionally accountable for developing, evaluating, and improving his or her own practices

Figure 2-2. Orientation Checklist

ORIENTATION CHECKLIST FOR THE INFECTION PREVENTIONIST

Employee Name: _____   Date of Hire: _____

Item	Date Completed
ID badge	
Attendance at new employee general orientation	
Pre-employment health evaluation by Employee Health	
Review of job description	
Review of performance evaluation (90-day, annual)	
Use of phones and voicemail	
Use of beepers and paging system	
Computers:	
• Personal codes	
• Mainframe training program	
• E-mail and Internet systems	
• Personal computer training programs, as needed	
Safety Issues:	
• Nearest fire exits and alarms	
• Emergency numbers	
• Right-to-know (MSDS)	
• Emergency Preparedness Manual and infection prevention responsibilities	
Joint Commission standards (Including list of standards and National Patient Safety Goals applicable to IPC)	
Hospital-wide policies and procedures (Hospital P&P Manual)	
Department policies and procedures (IPC Department P&P Manual)	
CDC guidelines	
APIC guidelines	
OSHA regulations	
• Bloodborne pathogens	
• Tuberculosis	
State regulations for IPC program	
Mandatory reporting requirements	
• State	
• Centers for Medicare & Medicaid Services (CMS)	
• Other	

(continued)

Figure 2-2. Orientation Checklist (continued)

Item	Date Completed
Communicable disease reporting:	
• Regulations	
• Report forms (TB, AIDS, STD, communicable diseases)	
Surveillance methodology:	
• Health care–associated infection (HAI) criteria	
• Data collection forms	
• Microbiology reports	
• Surveillance indicators for current year	
• Review of monthly reports/quarterly reports	
Surveillance activities:	
• Rounds and patient/resident chart review with IPC staff	
• Evaluation of patient/resident chart review done alone	
Preparing HAI report(s):	
• Sources of numerator data	
• Sources of denominator data	
• Tabulation of data	
• Preparing and distributing report(s)	
Infection Prevention and Control Committee:	
• Preparing agenda and attachments	
• Writing minutes	
Methodology for Policy and Procedure Review:	
• IC department P&P	
• Hospitalwide P&P	
• Department-specific P&P	
Committee attendance:	
• List of committees, including performance improvement activities	
• Duties/responsibilities for each	

This figure shows a checklist organizations should consider using to ensure a comprehensive orientation program for an infection preventionist. MSDS, material safety data sheet; IPC, infection prevention and control; P&P, policies and procedures; CDC, Centers for Disease Control and Prevention; APIC, Association for Professionals in Infection Control and Epidemiology; OSHA, Occupational Safety and Health Administration; TB, tuberculosis; STD, sexually transmitted disease; IC, infection control.

Source: Adapted from Arias K.: Personnel and nonpersonnel issues. In Arias K.: *Assessing and Developing an Infection Control Program in the Acute Care Setting*, 2nd ed. Washington, DC: Association for Professionals in Infection Control and Epidemiology, 2005, pp. C7-12–C7-13. Used with permission.

during this orientation.) In addition, a new infection preventionist should attend a basic training course in infection prevention and control within the first six months of beginning the position.

- *Designate responsibility for managing infection prevention and control activities within the organization.* A major responsibility of an infection preventionist is to coordinate and oversee the many infection prevention and control activities that occur within an organization. Most of these activities take place during direct patient care or while providing support services. Although it is not possible for an infection preventionist to directly observe, for example, whether each care provider is performing hand hygiene appropriately, cleaning and disinfecting equipment according to policy, or appropriately screening any visitors who may present a risk to patients, infection preventionists must ensure that clear policies and procedures exist to provide guidance for best practices and ensure that the staff and patients or residents are aware of these policies and are performing the required activities consistently.

To coordinate the infection prevention and control activities, an infection preventionist must develop partnerships and obtain the cooperation of point-of-care staff members who will accept the responsibility for implementing infection prevention and control efforts in their area. Although the infection preventionist delegates responsibility to these persons for infection prevention and control, managers should assign accountability to these persons to ensure that the IPC efforts are being carried out. This collaboration can be accomplished through sharing reports and data and encouraging communication between the point-of-care staff, managers, and the infection preventionist.

Coordination improves when there is multidisciplinary participation in the IPC program, such as when there is broad representation on an infection prevention and control committee or an infection prevention and control advisory council and direct communication with nursing councils and patient safety and performance improvement committees. An infection preventionist must have access to, and participate in, the work of these groups to facilitate communication throughout the organization. (*See* Sidebar 2-3 on page 12.)

- *Allocate appropriate staffing.* As previously mentioned, the staffing of an IPC program cannot be tied to bed size alone. The number and skill mix of personnel assigned to manage the program should be determined by the following organizational characteristics:
  — Scope of services
  — Procedures and treatments provided
  — Characteristics of the populations served
  — Geographic location
  — Organizational needs and complexity
  — Requirements and expectations of external agencies
  — Availability of nonpersonnel resources (such as computers, information technology, and laboratory support) required for performing essential activities

No nationally recognized standard for staffing IPC programs currently exists in the United States; however, several studies and reports have attempted to quantify the issue. As discussed earlier, the SENIC Project linked the availability of 1 infection preventionist per 250 occupied hospital beds with an effective hospital IPC program.[4] However, in 1996, the SHEA Consensus Panel noted that, for the hospital setting, "the old ratio of one infection control professional infection control professional (ICP) per 250 beds is no longer adequate, because the notion of a ratio tied to beds is now insufficient to define the scope of the work of an ICP."[11] A similar consensus panel was established by APIC and SHEA in 1997 to develop recommendations for optimal infrastructure and essential activities of infection control and epidemiology programs in out-of-hospital settings.[12] This panel noted that the IPC program must be "the responsibility of at least one designated person. In some health care organizations, this person may also have other responsibilities (that is, infection control activities will be part time). In this situation, the expected number of hours per week that are devoted to infection control should be clearly stated."[12]

In a 2002 infection prevention and control staffing study, a Delphi panel analyzed infection preventionist tasks and responsibilities in a variety of health care settings in the United States and estimated staffing levels for an appropriate IPC program.[15] For all settings, the panel recommended at least twice the staffing level of the SENIC Project report, with a ratio

Sidebar 2-3: Tips for Working Effectively with Administration or Leadership to Improve Infection Prevention and Control Activities

1. Know the expectations associated with your job description.
2. Introduce yourself to the chief executive officer or president of the organization.
3. Align departmental goals with the organization's strategic plan.
4. Spend some time with someone in the finance department to understand the costs of health care–associated infections (HAIs).
5. Form collaborative relationships with directors and managers of clinical support departments, especially those who directly impact infection prevention and control activities, such as laboratory, respiratory care, and sterile processing.
6. Establish close working relationships with the directors and managers of support departments, such as environmental services, purchasing, and materials management, to promote easy exchange of ideas for process improvements related to infection prevention and control.
7. Provide regular updates to administration on the state of infection prevention and control activities in the organization, including raw numbers of infection as well as rates.
8. Attend all meetings and fulfill responsibilities associated with administrative appointments to committees and task forces.
9. Negotiate for increased financial support or positions, with data in hand on cost and opportunity savings associated with infection prevention.
10. Provide a brief, easy-to-read, and understandable annual report to administration on the infection rates in the facility or organization. Be sure to include cost savings associated with a decrease in infections, including opportunity costs.*
11. Establish a relationship based on mutual trust with the bedside caregivers and patient care managers because this is where the prevention and control activities take place.
12. Help remove barriers to change for managers who wish to look at new infection prevention and control products and methods to prevent and control infections.

*__Note:__ *For information on making a business case for infection prevention, refer to the article by Perencevich et al. in the "Additional Readings" section at the end of this chapter.*

__Source:__ Deanie Lancaster, R.N., B.S.N., M.H.S.A., C.I.C. Used with permission.

of 0.8 to 1.0 infection preventionists for every 100 occupied acute care beds.[15] One of the most important findings of the Delphi study was that competing responsibilities and limited resources prevented many of the participants from performing IPC program tasks that the panel considered essential. The major conclusion of the Delphi study was that "recommendations for staffing must not only consider the number of occupied beds (average daily census) but also include the scope of the program, the complexity of the health care facility or system, the characteristics of the patient population, and the unique or urgent needs of the facility and community."[15]

In September 2008, the Ontario Ministry of Health and Long-Term Care Public Health Division/Provincial Infectious Diseases Advisory Committee, Toronto, issued *Best Practices for Infection Prevention and Control Programs in Ontario in All Health Care Settings.*[16] Similar to the previously mentioned reports and studies, this document notes that staffing should not be based exclusively on bed numbers and that the ratio of infection preventionists "will vary according to the acuity and activity of the health care facility and the volume and complexity"[16] of the infection preventionist's work. The committee provides the following recommendations for staffing and resources in Ontario health care facilities:

— A minimum ratio of 1.0 full-time-equivalent (FTE) infection preventionist per 115 acute care beds
— A minimum ratio of 1.0 FTE infection preventionist per 100 occupied acute care beds if there are high-risk activities (for example, dialysis)
— An additional ratio of 1.0 FTE infection

preventionist per 30 intensive care beds where ventilation and hemodynamic monitoring are routinely performed

— 1.0 FTE infection preventionist per 150 occupied long term care beds where there are ventilated patients, patients with spinal cord injuries, and patients undergoing dialysis or other high-acuity activities

— 1.0 FTE infection preventionist per 150–200 beds in other settings, depending on acuity levels[16]

As mentioned throughout this chapter, the ultimate responsibility for managing an IPC program should be assigned to one person. However, in many cases, especially in long term care facilities and small organizations, the person who manages the IPC program also oversees related areas, such as employee health, staff development, nursing, and performance improvement. In some settings, such as office-based practices or very small hospitals, it may be cost-effective to contract out all or some IPC functions, such as staff education and training, employee health, and exposure follow-up. Some organizations have successfully used infection control liaisons in a variety of health care settings to assist with IPC activities.[17]

No matter what the size and scope of an organization, its leaders and the person responsible for developing and maintaining the IPC program must collaborate to identify resource capabilities and match them with the organization's needs and external requirements. They must prioritize the infection preventionist's infection surveillance, prevention, and control activities and streamline work processes to increase efficiency. In some cases, it might be necessary to contract for IPC functions, share staff with other areas, transfer some responsibilities to other services or departments, or identify activities that are not essential.

TIP: *No matter what the size and scope of an organization, its leaders and the person responsible for developing and maintaining the IPC program must collaborate to identify resource capabilities and match them with the organization's needs and external requirements. They must prioritize the infection preventionist's infection surveillance, prevention, and control activities and streamline work processes to increase efficiency.*

RELATED STANDARDS

In addition to Standard IC.01.01.01, several standards throughout the *Comprehensive Accreditation Manuals* relate to allocating effective resources to an IPC program. The following sections take a look at two relevant standards.

Standard HR.01.02.01, EP 1: The [organization] defines staff qualifications specific to their job responsibilities. *Note 2:* Qualifications for infection control may be met through ongoing education, training, experience, and/or certification (such as that offered by the Certification Board of Infection Control and Epidemiology).

As previously mentioned, the person(s) assigned to manage an IPC program should meet certain core competencies. The organization's leadership should recognize and support learning opportunities and the need for the infection preventionist's ongoing education. The health care field and the practice of infection prevention and control are rapidly evolving. To ensure that an infection preventionist's knowledge remains current, leadership should make provisions that allow the infection preventionist to attend professional meetings and educational programs, access information through the Internet and other resources, purchase relevant textbooks and publications, and take the infection control certification examination.[14] (*See* Chapter 3.)

LD.02.01.01, EP 3: Leaders communicate the mission, vision, and goals to staff and the population the organization serves.

An organization's leaders are expected to demonstrate support of the IPC program. This can be accomplished by discussing and supporting hand hygiene compliance, multidrug-resistant organism (MDRO) management, and bundles and other infection prevention strategies in management meetings, during leadership rounds, in high-level committee meetings, and in the organization's newsletter.

Clinical leaders can express support and serve as role models by incorporating infection prevention practices into their daily activities.[18] For example, studies have shown that hand hygiene compliance in health care workers increases when a physician leader, such as the medical director of an intensive care unit making rounds with residents, routinely practices good hand hygiene and expects his or her team to do likewise.[18]

Taking Responsibility for Preventing and Controlling Infections

Although the responsibility for *managing* an IPC program is assigned to a few individuals, all health care providers are responsible for *using* appropriate infection prevention practices in their daily activities. Both the "Infection Prevention and Control" and "Human Resources" standards address this topic.

STANDARD IC.01.05.01

EP 6: All hospital and critical access hospital components and functions are integrated into infection prevention and control activities. (*See also* HR.01.04.01, EPs 2 and 4.) *Note:* for home care, ambulatory care, long term care, and behavioral care, IC.01.05.01, EP 6, is stated as follows: Everyone who works in the organization has responsibilities for preventing and controlling infection.

STANDARD HR.01.04.01

EP 2: The [organization] orients its staff to the key safety content before staff provide care, treatment, and services. Completion of this orientation is documented.

STANDARD HR.01.04.01

EP 4: The [organization] orients staff on the following: Their specific job duties, including those related to infection prevention and control and assessing and managing pain. Completion of this orientation is documented.

Standard IC.01.05.01, EP 6, requires health care organizations to educate personnel about their specific roles and responsibilities in infection prevention and control. Standard HR.01.04.01, EPs 2 and 4 require that organizations provide orientation training related to infection prevention and control to all staff. Based on these requirements, the organization's leadership is expected both to educate staff members on their responsibilities regarding infection prevention and control and to hold staff members accountable for adhering to appropriate infection prevention and control practices.

SUMMARY

The goal of an IPC program is to reduce the occurrence of HAIs to the lowest possible levels. Regardless of the health care setting, and infection surveillance, prevention, and control program should be managed by an individual or individuals who have prescribed core competencies. The types and number of personnel and other resources allocated should be based on the organization's size, type, and complexity and on an assessment of the populations served, services provided, and internal and external requirements. The organization's leaders should ensure that appropriate resources are allocated to establish and maintain an IPC program that effectively reduces the risk and occurrence of HAIs. Although the responsibility for managing the IPC program is assigned to a few individuals, everyone who works in a health care organization has responsibilities for preventing and controlling infections.

FURTHER RESOURCES

The following sections provide further information on this topic and can serve as a valuable reference in allocating resources to an IPC program.

CD Tool

Tool 2-1: Infection Control Director Position Description/Evaluation—Sky Ridge Medical Center

Web Sites

- Association for Professionals in Infection Control and Epidemiology: http://www.apic.org
- Centers for Disease Control and Prevention, Division of Healthcare Quality Promotion (DHQP): http://www.cdc.gov/ncidod/dhqp/index.html
- Society for Healthcare Epidemiology of America: http://www.shea-online.org

Additional Readings

- Association for Professionals in Infection Control and Epidemiology (APIC): *APIC Text of Infection Control and Epidemiology*, 3rd ed. Washington, DC: APIC, 2009.
- Friedman C., et al.: APIC/CHICA–Canada infection prevention, control, and epidemiology: Professional and practice standards. *Am J Infect Control* 36:385–389, Aug. 2008. Available at http://www.apic.org/ Content/NavigationMenu/PracticeGuidance/ APICCHICAStandards/APIC_CHICA_Standards.pdf.

- Friedman C., et al.: Requirements for infrastructure and essential activities of infection control and epidemiology in out-of-hospital settings: A Consensus Panel report. *Am J Infect Control* 27:418–430, Oct. 1999. Available at http://www.apic.org/AM/ Template.cfm?Section=Search&section=Consensus_ Reports&template=/CM/ContentDisplay.cfm& ContentFileID=277.

- Lee T.B., et al.: Recommended practices for surveillance: Association for Professionals in Infection Control and Epidemiology (APIC), Inc. *Am J Infect Control* 5:427–440, Sep. 2007. Available at http://www.apic.org/Content/NavigationMenu/ PracticeGuidance/SurveillanceDefinitionsReportsand Recommendations/AJIC_Surveillance_2007.pdf.

- Perencevich E.N., et al.: Raising standards while watching the bottom line: Making a business case for infection control. *Infect Control Hosp Epidemiol* 28:1121–1133, 2007.

- Scheckler W.E., et al.: Requirements for infrastructure and essential activities of infection control and epidemiology in hospitals: A Consensus Panel report. *Am J Infect Control* 26:47–60, Feb. 1998. Available at http://www.apic.org/AM/Template.cfm?Section= Search&section=Consensus_Reports&template=/CM/ ContentDisplay.cfm&ContentFileID=284.

- Smith P.W., et al.: SHEA/APIC Guideline: Infection Prevention and Control in the Long-Term Care Facility. *Infect Control Hosp Epidemiol* 29:785–814, Sep. 2008. Available at http://www.journals.uchicago.edu/ doi/pdf/10.1086/592416.

- Stone P.W., et al.: Staffing and structure of infection prevention and control programs. *Am J Infect Control* 37:351–357, 2009.

REFERENCES

1. Klevens R.M., et al.: Estimating health care–associated infections and deaths in U.S. hospitals, 2002. *Public Health Rep* 122:160–166, Mar.–Apr. 2007.
2. Burke J.P.: Infection control—A problem for patient safety. *N Engl J Med* 348:651–656, Feb. 13, 2003.
3. Harbarth S., Sax H., Gastmeier R.: The preventable proportion of nosocomial infections: An overview of published reports. *J Hosp Infect* 54:258–266, Aug. 2003.
4. Haley R.W., et al.: The efficacy of infection surveillance and control programs in preventing nosocomial infections in U.S. hospitals. *Am J Epidemiol* 121:182–205, Feb. 1985.
5. Centers for Disease Control and Prevention: Monitoring hospital-acquired infections to promote patient safety—United States, 1990–1999. *MMWR Morb Mortal Wkly Rep* 49:149–153, Mar. 10, 2000.
6. Muto C., et al.: Reduction in central line–associated bloodstream infections among patients in intensive care units—Pennsylvania, April 2001–March 2005. *MMWR Morb Mortal Wkly Rep* 54:1013–1016, Oct. 14, 2005.
7. Pronovost P., et al.: An intervention to decrease catheter-related bloodstream infections in the ICU. *N Engl J Med* 355:2725–2732, Dec. 2006.
8. Jarvis W.R.: Infection control and changing health-care delivery systems. *Emerg Infect Dis* 7:170–173, Mar.–Apr. 2001.
9. Goldrick B.A.: The practice of infection control and applied epidemiology: A historical perspective. *Am J Infect Control* 33:493–500, Nov. 2005.
10. Hass J.P.: Measurement of infection control department performance: State of the science. *Am J Infect Control* 34:543–549, Nov. 2006.
11. Scheckler W.E., et al.: Requirements for infrastructure and essential activities of infection control and epidemiology in hospitals: A Consensus Panel report. *Am J Infect Control* 26:47–60, Feb. 1998.
12. Friedman C., et al.: Requirements for infrastructure and essential activities of infection control and epidemiology in out-of-hospital settings: A Consensus Panel report. *Am J Infect Control* 27:418–430, Oct. 1999.
13. Friedman C., et al.: APIC/CHICA–Canada infection prevention, control, and epidemiology: Professional and practice standards. *Am J Infect Control* 36:385–389, Aug. 2008.
14. Certification Board of Infection Control and Epidemiology, Inc.: *Home page.* http://www.cbic.org (accessed Feb. 6, 2009).
15. O'Boyle C.O., Jackson M., Henly S.J.: Staffing requirements for infection control programs in US health care facilities: Delphi project. *Am J Infect Control* 30:321–333, Oct. 2002.
16. Ontario Ministry of Health and Long-Term Care Public Health Division/Provincial Infectious Diseases Advisory Committee: *Best Practices for Infection Prevention and Control Programs in Ontario in All Health Care Settings.* Sep. 2008. http://www.health.gov.on.ca/english/providers/program/infectious /diseases/best_prac/bp_ipcp_20080905.pdf (accessed Feb. 6, 2009).
17. Wright J., et al.: Expanding the infection control team: Development of the infection control liaison position for the neonatal intensive care unit. *Am J Infect Control* 30:174–178, May 2002.
18. Lankford M.G., et al.: Influence of role models and hospital design on hand hygiene of health care workers. *Emerg Infect Dis* 9:21–223, Feb. 2003.

Chapter 3

The Role of Leadership in Infection Prevention and Control Programs

Russell N. Olmsted, M.P.H., C.I.C.; and Barbara Moore Soule, R.N., M.P.A., C.I.C.

It is critical for leaders of an organization to be aware and supportive of the infection prevention and control (IPC) program to ensure that it is effective and contributes to an environment and culture of patient safety. However, leadership involvement in infection prevention and control activities varies in different organizations. For example, the results of a survey of almost 1,000 health professionals, including those in the fields of quality, patient safety, and infection prevention and control—conducted by the Association for Professionals in Infection Control and Epidemiology (APIC) and Premier Inc. Healthcare Alliance in 2008—revealed some notable gaps in the engagement of organization leadership in IPC programs.[1] Consider the following statistics from this study:

- Only 15% of survey respondents indicated that executive and physician leaderships are actively engaged and leading the charge against infections in their facilities.
- Only 30.3% suggested that executives and physicians are the most important resource in meeting challenges related to health care–associated infections (HAIs).
- Although almost 60% indicated that HAI data are shared with executive leaders and boards of directors, only 15% indicated that feedback is provided from these leaders to the infection prevention and control and patient safety professionals.

This same survey identified opportunities for improvement that included the need for the following:

- Specific calls to action from physician and administrative leadership to elevate the priority level of HAI prevention
- Incorporating methods for regularly sharing HAI surveillance findings with executive leaders

- A team approach focusing on earlier identification of HAIs and implementation of infection-prevention interventions
- Sufficient resources and support from administration and other hospital staff to implement a system of continuous performance evaluation and quality and patient safety improvements

LEADERS INFLUENCE THE PERFORMANCE OF THE INFECTION PREVENTION AND CONTROL PROGRAM

Although most leaders will not be directly involved in the day-to-day operations of an IPC program, the decisions they make and the initiatives they implement will affect the program and outcomes of care. In other words, the actions of leadership have a direct and critical impact on the performance of the IPC program.

As previously mentioned, a comprehensive and effective IPC program is a critical component of a safety- and quality-based culture. The Joint Commission has identified the following key systems that influence the effective performance of an organization with regard to establishing and supporting a culture of safety and quality (*see also* Figure 3-1 on page 18):

- Using data
- Planning
- Communicating
- Changing performance
- Staffing

These systems are like pillars, rooted in the foundation set by leadership and supporting the many organizationwide processes, such as infection prevention, that are important to

Figure 3-1. The Five Pillars of Effective Performance

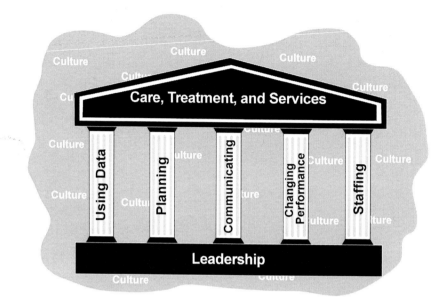

This figure illustrates the role of leadership in the performance of the five pillars that contribute to a culture of safety and quality.

Source: The Joint Commission.

"INFECTION PREVENTION AND CONTROL" (IC) STANDARDS

Standard IC.01.02.01

[Organization] leaders allocate needed resources for the infection prevention and control program.

"LEADERSHIP" (LD) STANDARDS

Standard LD.01.03.01

The governing body is ultimately accountable for the safety and quality of care.

Standard LD.02.01.01

The mission, vision, and goals of the [organization] support the safety and quality of care, treatment, and services.

Standard LD.03.01.01

Leaders create and maintain a culture of safety and quality throughout the [organization].

Standard LD.03.02.01

The [organization] uses data and information to guide decisions and to understand variation in the performance of processes supporting safety and quality.

Standard LD.03.03.01

Leaders use [organization]-wide planning to establish structures and processes that focus on safety and quality.

Standard LD.03.04.01

The [organization] communicates information related to safety and quality to those who need it, including staff, licensed independent practitioners, [patients], families, and external interested parties.

Standard LD.03.05.01

Leaders implement changes in existing processes to improve the performance of the [organization].

Standard LD.03.06.01

Those who work in the [organization] are focused on improving safety and quality.

individual care, treatment, and services. These systems inter-relate and work together to support safe, high-quality care. Permeating this entire structure is the culture of the organization. The effective performance of these systems results in a culture in which safety and quality are priorities.

This chapter discusses leadership in the context of a culture of safety and each of the five leadership systems supported by both the "Infection Prevention and Control" (IC) and "Leadership" (LD) standards. Although this chapter provides an introduction to the relevant LD standards, the reader is encouraged to carefully review the entire leadership chapter and consider how the standards relate to the IPC program.

TIP: *Although most leaders will not be directly involved in the day-to-day operations of an IPC program, the decisions they make and the initiatives they implement will affect the program and outcomes of care.*

EXPLORING THE LEADERSHIP STANDARDS RELATED TO INFECTION PREVENTION AND CONTROL

As previously mentioned, this chapter addresses selected standards in the IC and LD chapters that apply to the role of leadership in the IPC program. The following sections take a brief look at these standards.

LD.02.01.01: The mission, vision, and goals of the [organization] support the safety and quality of care, treatment, and services.

The organization's mission, vision, and goals should delineate how it will promote safety and quality, including how it will promote infection prevention and control. Because the organization's goals are focused on improving the quality of care and achieving the best outcomes for all patients and residents, regardless of where health care is delivered, it is important that the organization's leaders support the IPC program's goals, objectives, and strategies for preventing infections. (For more information on specific prevention strategies, *see* Chapter 6.) Barbara Farrell, director, Quality and Innovation, American Organization of Nurse Executives, captured the essence of aligning the mission, vision, and goals of an organization with prevention of infection by observing that infection prevention needs to engage not only from the top—the board and executive leadership—down, but also from the

frontline caregiver up, adding that "that's the best way to get input and ownership. Patients need to be involved as well."[2]

TIP: *Because the organization's goals are focused on improving the quality of care and achieving best outcomes for all patients and residents, regardless of where health care is delivered, it is important that the organization's leaders support the IPC program's goals, objectives, and strategies for preventing infections.*

LD.03.01.01: Leaders create and maintain a culture of safety throughout the organization.

The individual and aggregate beliefs, attitudes, and values of leaders and staff create the culture of an organization and influence how effectively the organization performs. This extends to the IPC program. One of the hallmarks of a culture of patient safety is that all persons wish to achieve and maintain excellence and to eliminate harm to patients and staff. Personal responsibility is accepted and widespread. For IPC programs, these attitudes are essential if infection risks are to be minimized and infections prevented.

An organization demonstrates compliance with this standard when leaders create a culture of patient safety by insisting on teamwork and accountability to reduce the risk of adverse events, such as infections. Infection preventionists can support this philosophy by working with teams of caregivers to enhance best practices, such as by providing bundled care practices to reduce central line–associated bloodstream infection (CLABSI) or ventilator-associated pneumonia. The safe-culture philosophy promotes systems that target the elimination of HAIs, support open discussions about infections that do occur, and encourage reporting of infection issues.

As infection preventionists work collaboratively with staff, they should note that improving processes of care involves looking at system breakdowns and not blaming individuals when infections occur, unless there has been obvious disregard for observing approved infection prevention practices.

LD.03.02.01: The organization uses data and information to guide decisions and to understand variation in the performance of processes supporting quality and safety.

STANDARD LD.03.02.01

EP 1: Leaders set expectations for using data and information to improve the safety and quality of care, treatment, and services.

EP 4: Leaders provide the resources needed for data and information use, including staff, equipment, and information systems.

EP 5: The organization uses data and information in decision making that supports the safety and quality of care, treatment, and services.

EP 6: The organization uses data and information to identify and respond to internal and external changes in the environment.

An important responsibility of organization leaders is to make informed decisions about patient care and staff safety relative to infection prevention. For these decisions, leaders must have valid and reliable data about clinical processes and outcomes, as well as financial information. Leaders should set the expectation that data are integral to managing care and should provide the resources to obtain, analyze, and use information to maintain best practices and achieve change when necessary.

Leaders often need to receive financial data to factor into overall patient care and staff safety decisions. They increasingly request that infection preventionists make the business case with return on investment (ROI) for a new procedure, supplies or equipment, or infrastructure changes. (For information on making a business case for infection prevention, refer to the article by Perencevich et al. in the "Additional Readings" section at the end of this chapter.)

Despite leaders' focus on using data to make decisions, important gaps remain in understanding the economics of HAIs as well as in accessing, collating, and using critical data related to these infections. Two recent surveys identified that although infection preventionists spend more than 40% of their time conducting surveillance, the use and penetration of information technology to enhance efficiency of the surveillance activity is lacking.[3,4] Consequently, to better serve the organization and to receive accurate and timely data, it is important for leaders to assess and enhance use of information technology within the IPC program. To improve the use of such technology and to meet Joint Commission requirements, an organization's leaders should provide the following to the IPC program and staff[5]:

- *Computer workstation and internal network connectivity.* These are essential for access to data needed for surveillance of HAIs, such as information on a patient's or resident's treatment, diagnostic test results, and therapy provided. Access requires connectivity to patient, pharmacy, and laboratory information systems (LIS); imaging studies; and admission/discharge/transfer (ADT) information.

Computer applications that increase efficiency and automation of the steps involved in the surveillance of HAIs are also available. One example is a data-mining program that merges databases such as the ADT, LIS, and pharmacy databases to identify patients and patterns that warrant additional review by the infection preventionist. The cost benefits of such programs have recently been analyzed. The findings indicate that, although useful, many of these programs require a considerable investment.[6-9]

Additional benefits have been and are going to be realized as health systems and providers move toward the use of an electronic health record (EHR). Researchers have identified potential for the EHR to support infection prevention and control surveillance, such as in its application for automated collection of device days.[10,11] Infection preventionists and organization leaders need to weigh the costs and benefits of these systems for their program and determine a prudent, fiscally responsible course.

- *Computer program applications.* These include word-processing, data collection/analysis, and presentation programs, as well as Internet and intranet connectivity that provide access to health information, such as bibliographic search engines, online textbooks, and journals.

- *Computer-based system for surveillance and management of critical data and information.* With the significant growth in federal and state-based mandates for disclosure of facility-specific HAI data, organization leaders should consider supporting enrollment of their IPC programs in a broadly used and tested database program. One such program used by many facilities is the Centers for Disease Control and Prevention's (CDC's) National Healthcare Safety Network (NHSN). The NHSN is a secure, Internet-based application that facilitates use of HAI surveillance definitions and methods, provides a national platform for purposes of estimating magnitude and trends of HAIs, offers risk-adjusted data for intra- and inter-facility comparison, and serves as a collaborative performance improvement network.[12] Many states require use of the NHSN for mandatory reporting programs.[3] Other surveillance programs that use clinical document architecture (CDA) standards issued by the CDC and commercial programs can be used for meeting IPC program needs and public reporting requirements.

■ *Communications networks.* Electronic communication networks that use e-mail, rich site summary (RSS), and other systems to distribute information and electronic alerts from professional organizations, public health agencies, and other government agencies provide an infection preventionist and an organization's leaders with up-to-date information on applicable standards, guidelines, regulations, outbreaks, product recalls, and emerging infectious diseases. The organization should provide Internet access to the infection preventionist and other organization leaders so they can identify applicable networks and subscribe to their services.

TIP: *Leaders should set the expectation that data are integral to managing care and should provide the resources to obtain, analyze, and use information to maintain best practices and achieve change when necessary.*

Standard IC.01.02.01 Also Addresses Resources and Information

The LD standards address the overall concept of using data and information to drive safety, and Standard IC.01.02.01 discusses the topic as it relates to infection prevention and control. Specifically, the standard requires organizations to allocate resources and provide access to information needed to support IPC efforts.

Standard IC.01.02.01: [Organization] leaders allocate needed resources for the infection prevention and control program.

EP 1: The [organization] provides access to information needed to support the infection prevention and control program.

EP 2: The [organization] provides laboratory resources when needed to support the infection prevention and control program.

EP 3: The [organization] provides equipment and supplies to support the infection prevention and control program.

The second element of performance (EP) for Standard IC.01.02.01 requires infection preventionists to have access to the LIS to perform their responsibilities. Access can be accomplished by generating and providing the infection preventionist with a routine LIS report, either electronically or in hard copy. The availability of data-mining and other information technology tools also can be identified as evidence of compliance with this EP.

Organizations that use reference laboratories should have immediate access to the data necessary not only to diagnose and treat infections but also to allow the infection preventionist to put in place prevention and control methods as quickly as possible. Policies should be implemented with these laboratories to require immediate notification of significant results associated with communicable diseases and epidemiologically significant organisms, such as methicillin-resistant *Staphylococcus aureus* (MRSA) or *Clostridium difficile*. These policies can be negotiated by smaller facilities, including long term care facilities, as part of the contract with the reference laboratory. Of note, many smaller acute care and long term care facilities contract with commercial third-party clinical laboratories. Leaders in these organizations need to ensure that infection preventionists have full access to LIS reports and periodic analysis of microbiologic data, such as susceptibility profiles, from these third-party laboratories.

TIP: *Leaders should insist that infection preventionists provide input when new or updated laboratory systems are being considered, especially in microbiology. This will provide an opportunity to shape the data generation and reports that are most helpful to the organization.*

The third EP of Standard IC.01.02.01, which addresses equipment and supplies, requires leaders to ensure that the organization's infrastructure supports other nonpersonnel resources needed for an effective IPC program.[5] These resources include office space, associated equipment (printer, fax machine, pager, telephone, and so on), and printing services. In addition, to meet this EP, provisions should be made to provide reference books and journals for the infection preventionist; printed materials for patient, resident, visitor, family, and staff education; and computers to prepare educational materials and presentations.

Evidence of leadership support for resource allocation also can be demonstrated by the availability of other supplies and equipment needed to sustain the IPC program. These may include the following:

- Hand hygiene products
- Personal protective equipment (PPE)
- Sharps devices with engineered safety features
- Cleaning/disinfection/sterilization products and equipment
- Device trays/kits containing materials to promote aseptic technique
- Vaccines for patients, residents, and personnel

For a checklist of resources needed for an effective IPC program, *see* CD Tool 3-1, "Resources for an Infection Prevention and Control Program."

LD.03.03.01: Leaders use organization-wide planning to establish structures and processes that focus on safety and quality.

> **STANDARD LD.03.03.01**
>
> EP 1: Planning activities focus on improving patient safety and health care quality.
>
> EP 5: Safety and quality planning is organization-wide.
>
> EP 6: Planning activities adapt to changes in the environment.

Organizationwide planning is essential to support the functions of the IPC program. Organizations can demonstrate compliance with this standard—with regard to infection prevention and control—when there is evidence that leaders have included the IPC team in the planning of patient safety and quality activities and goals. An infection preventionist should work to secure a seat at the planning table as part of a multidisciplinary team and to provide the organization with pertinent information about trends in infection prevention and control, emerging pathogens and diseases, new regulations, infectious diseases in community populations, and other issues that affect patient care and safety. An organization's leadership should be aware that infection preventionists play a critical role in providing information that can guide planning activities needed to respond to changes in the environment, such as a potential influx of patients and staff shortages due to pandemic influenza.

LD.03.04.01: The [organization] communicates information related to safety and quality to those who need it, including staff, licensed independent practitioners, [patients], families and external interested parties.

> **STANDARD LD.03.04.01**
>
> EP 1: Communication processes foster the safety of the patient and the quality of care.
>
> EP 3: Communication is designed to meet the needs of internal and external users.
>
> EP 4: Leaders provide the resources required for communication, based on the needs of patients, the community, physicians, staff, and management.

To meet this standard in the context of infection prevention and control, leaders must ensure that systems are in place to communicate relevant information about infection issues, processes, and outcomes and that this communication is available to staff, patients or residents, visitors, and volunteers throughout the organization in a timely and understandable fashion. In addition, communication efforts must also include mechanisms for the IPC program to successfully and easily communicate with external groups that collect infection-related data, statistics, and events, such as the state health department (for reportable infections) and quality improvement agencies (for HAI reporting requirements). Strategies for internal and external communication are discussed in Chapter 7.

LD.03.05.01: Leaders implement changes in existing processes to improve the performance of the organization.

> **STANDARD LD.03.05.01**
>
> EP 3: The organization has a systematic approach to change and performance improvement.
>
> EP 4: Leaders provide the resources required for performance improvement and change management including sufficient staff, access to information, and training.

Creating change, improving performance, and sustaining improvement are more likely to be successful with strong leadership commitment, role modeling, and a proactive, systematic, and collaborative approach. Leaders must provide adequate resources for performance improvement teams and must allot time for projects to ensure effective, sustained improvement. A strong, visible emphasis on the culture of safety throughout an organization will provide the foundation for adherence to effective prevention practices and continuous performance improvement. (*See* CD Tool 3-2: "Methods for Leadership Support of Infection Prevention and Control Activities.")

In this context, organization change agents need to include a wide range of disciplines, including affiliated physicians. Saint et al. have published findings from a mixed-methods, representative nationwide survey of hospitals' adoption of evidence-based infection prevention interventions,[13,14] in which clinical champions, especially those representing

nursing and physicians, were found to be very effective agents for change in practices that improve performance. The converse was also identified; there are both personnel and organizational attributes that inhibit adoption of new evidence-based practices or changes in work practices. [14] (*See* Case Study 3-1, below, which describes a successful collaborative to reduce CLABSIs and the leadership support that helped make the collaborative successful. This example describes significant involvement of physician champions, such as intensivists. *See also* CD Tool 3-3, "Checklist of Methods to Involve Physicians in Infection Prevention and Control Activities," for ways to involve physician champions in the IPC program.)

Case Study 3-1. Saint Joseph Mercy Health System Experience: Keystone Intensive Care Unit Collaborative and Central Line–Associated Bloodstream Infection

Saint Joseph Mercy Health System (SJMHS) is a regional integrated health care delivery network located in southeastern Michigan. Two of its divisions—a 529-bed community teaching hospital and a 136-bed community hospital—participated in a statewide performance improvement project sponsored by the Michigan Health and Hospital Association called Keystone Intensive Care Unit (K-ICU). All four ICUs at these two facilities enrolled in the K-ICU.

The K-ICU collaborative was supported by a grant from the Agency for Healthcare Research and Quality (AHRQ), and the principal investigator was Dr. Peter Pronovost.[15] The primary aim of this research project was to combine scientific evidence of several effective, but separate, strategies for preventing CLABSI into a prevention "bundle" or composite. These strategies included the following five interventions:
- Hand hygiene
- Preparation of the insertion site with chlorhexidine gluconate
- Use of maximal sterile barrier precautions by the person inserting the line
- Avoidance of the femoral vein for insertion
- Daily assessment for continued need plus prompt removal of the central line

The K-ICU collaborative was remarkably successful both at SJMHS and at all other participating facilities. More than 100 ICUs in 77 hospitals enrolled in the collaborative, which began in early 2004. After an 18-month period of using the prevention bundle, participants showed a 66% reduction in the rate of CLABSI (the mean rate at baseline was 7.7 CLABSIs/1,000 central line days, which dropped to 1.4 CLABSIs/1,000 central line days by the 18-month mark).[15] This success has been sustained to the extent that through 2008 an estimated 1,800 lives had been saved, 129,000 excess days had been conserved, and $247 million in health care expenditures had been avoided.[16]

One ICU at the 136-bed hospital in SJMHS has gone for more than three years without a CLABSI, and the ICUs at the larger hospital all have seen no CLABSIs for periods of 8–12 months.

Infection preventionists participated as key members of K-ICU teams by providing the outcome data; however, the major emphasis of this study was on development of effective interdisciplinary collaboration by personnel in the ICUs. For example, education, supplies, equipment, and real-time performance monitoring and feedback systems

(continued)

Case Study 3-1. Saint Joseph Mercy Health System Experience: Keystone Intensive Care Unit Collaborative and Central Line–Associated Bloodstream Infection (continued)

---

were all coordinated by unit-based leadership. A transformation framework (*see* Sidebar 3-1, right), in combination with the Comprehensive Unit-based Safety Program (CUSP), was implemented to enhance communication and teamwork.

One tool that helped facilitate consistent and reliable delivery of the bundle elements was a checklist that the bedside nurse used in real time during the insertion of the central line by the physician. The Centers for Disease Control and Prevention's National Healthcare Safety Network offers the same process-monitoring tool in its Central Line Insertion Practices (CLIP) Module (available at http://www.cdc.gov/nhsn/forms/57.125_CLIP_BLANK.pdf).

A hallmark of the K-ICU success was engaged and visible leadership support for the collaborative from inception. This, plus a commitment to assessment and improvement of the culture of safety in the unit, was a key ingredient for success.

Sidebar 3-1. Framework for Transforming Evidence: The Four *E*'s

Engage: Personnel at the bedside, unit leadership, and organization leadership all need to be engaged in the project and the work of prevention.

Educate: The elements of the bundle need to be explained to providers who must be educated on their application.

Execute: Staff should implement the elements of the prevention bundle and ensure that they are used consistently.

Evaluate: Staff need to measure the impact of the new prevention bundle and provide these results back to the providers involved.

Source: Barbara M. Soule, R.N., M.P.A., C.I.C.

LD.03.06.01: Those who work in the [organization] are focused on improving safety and quality.

> **STANDARD LD.03.06.01**
> EP 3: Leaders provide for a sufficient number and mix of individuals to support safety, quality care, treatment, and services.
> EP 4: Those who work in the [organization] are competent to complete their assigned responsibilities.

The two EPs for LD.03.06.01 correlate with Standard IC.01.01.01 discussed in Chapter 2 and emphasize the leaders' responsibility to ensure that the infection prevention and control team is composed of adequate numbers of competent persons whose training and experience align with their responsibilities in the IPC program.

Leaders also have a responsibility to adequately staff the patient care team and the support groups to provide the highest quality of care. Although a thorough discussion of this topic is beyond the scope of this chapter, some studies have shown a relationship between understaffing and the occurrence of HAIs. Specifically, several studies have linked compromised staffing effectiveness, the skill mix of supplementary staffing, and breakdowns in culture of safety and work assignments with an increased risk of HAIs and other adverse outcomes affecting patient safety.[17–19]

SUMMARY

An organization's administrative, patient care, and clinical leadership play an essential role in supporting the activities of the IPC program. Several concepts regarding organization leadership involvement are reviewed in this chapter, including the following:

- Leadership should provide adequate resources to support patient safety and quality, including infection prevention and control. Gaps continue to exist between ideal resource levels for the IPC program and the current state.

- Both nonpersonnel resources, such as information technology, and personnel resources are essential tools for supporting the efficiency and effectiveness of an IPC program.

- Key leadership strategies directly influence infection

prevention and control practices. Such strategies include promoting a culture of safety and quality, using data and information to make patient care decisions, engaging in organizationwide planning for care, communicating about infection prevention and control issues, managing change and performance improvement to prevent infections, and providing adequate staffing to keep patients safe and to support the IPC program.

- Clinical champions from a variety of disciplines, such as nursing and physicians, are essential to realizing changes in work practices and improve the culture of safety. Organization leaders can facilitate engagement by identifying these champions and encouraging their support.

FURTHER RESOURCES

The following sections provide further information on this topic and can serve as valuable references in improving leadership involvement in IPC efforts.

CD Tools

Tool 3-1: Resources for an Infection Prevention and Control Program

Tool 3-2: Methods for Leadership Support of Infection Prevention and Control Activities

Tool 3-3: Checklist of Methods to Involve Physicians in Infection Prevention and Control Activities

Additional Readings

- Koll B.S., et al: The CLABs collaborative: A regionwide effort to improve the quality of care in hospitals. *Jt Comm J Qual Patient Saf* 34:713–723, Dec. 2008.
- Koteyko N., Carter R.: Discourse of "transformational leadership" in infection control. *Health (London)* 12:479–499, Oct. 2008.
- Larson E.L., et. al.: An organizational climate intervention associated with increased handwashing and decreased nosocomial infections. *Behav Med* 26:14–22, Spring 2000.
- Owens R.C.: *Clostridium difficile*–associated disease: Changing epidemiology and implications for management. *Drugs* 67:487–502, 2007.
- Perencevich E.N., et al.: Raising standards while

watching the bottom line: Making a business case for infection control. *Infect Control Hosp Epidemiol* 28:1121–1133, 2007.

- Pittet D., et. al.: Effectiveness of a hospital-wide programme to improve compliance with hand hygiene. *Lancet* 356:1307–1312, 2000.
- Stone P.W., et al.: Effect of guideline implementation on costs of hand hygiene. *Nurs Econ* 25:279–284, Sep.–Oct 2007.
- Warye K., Granato J.: Target: Zero hospital-acquired infections. *Healthc Financ Manage* 63:86–91, Jan. 2009.
- Weber S.G., Soule B.M.: *What Every Health Care Executive Should Know: The Cost of Antibiotic Resistance.* 2008. Available at http://www.jcrinc.com/MDRO-ToolKit/.

REFERENCES

1. Premier Inc.: *News Release: Survey Cites Executive and Physician Leadership, Adherence to Infection Prevention Practices as Areas of Improvement to Prevent Healthcare-Associated Infections, Improve Patient Care.* Sep. 23, 2008. http://www.premierinc.com/about/news/08-sep/APIC-premier-survey.jsp (accessed Mar. 9, 2009).
2. Arthur D., et al.: Hospital-acquired infections: Leadership challenges. Panel discussion. *Hosp Health Netw* 82:56–65, Oct. 2008.
3. Stricof R.L., et al.: Infection control resources in New York State hospitals, 2007. *Am J Infect Control* 36:702–705, Dec. 2008.
4. Stone P.W., et al.: Staffing and structure of infection prevention and control programs. *Am J Infect Control* 37:351–357, Jun. 2009.
5. Scheckler W.E., et al.: Requirements for infrastructure and essential activities of infection control and epidemiology in hospitals: A Consensus Panel report. *Am J Infect Control* 26:47–60, Feb. 2009.
6. Furuno J.P., et al.: Economics of infection control surveillance technology: Cost-effective or just cost? *Am J Infect Control* 36(3 Suppl.):S12–S17, Apr. 2008.
7. Dao T.K., et al.: A practical data mining method to link hospital microbiology and an infection control database. *Am J Infect Control* 36(3 Suppl.):S18–S20, Apr. 2008.
8. Young J., Stevenson K.B.: Real-time surveillance and decision support: Optimizing infection control and antimicrobial choices at the point of care. *Am J Infect Control* 36(3 Suppl.):S67–S74, Apr. 2008.
9. Trick W.: Building a data warehouse for infection control. *Am J Infect Control* 36(3 Suppl.):S67–S74, Apr. 2008.
10. Atreja A., et al.: Opportunities and challenges in utilizing electronic health records for infection surveillance, prevention, and control. *Am J Infect Control* 36(3 Suppl.):S67–S74, Apr. 2008.

11. Wright M.O., et al.: The electronic medical record as a tool for infection surveillance: Successful automation of device-days. *Am J Infect Control* 37:364–370, Jun. 2009.

12. Centers for Disease Control and Prevention: *National Healthcare Safety Network (NHSN)*. http://www.cdc.gov/nhsn/index.html (accessed Jun. 3, 2009).

13. Saint S., et al.: A multicenter qualitative study on preventing hospital-acquired urinary tract infection in US hospitals. *Infect Control Hosp Epidemiol* 29:333–341, Apr. 2008.

14. Saint S., et al: How active resisters and organizational constipators affect health care–acquired infection prevention efforts. *Jt Comm J Qual Patient Saf* 35:239–246, May 2009.

15. Pronovost P., et al.: An intervention to decrease catheter-related bloodstream infections in the ICU. *N Engl J Med* 355:2725–2732, Dec. 28, 2006.

16. Pronovost P.: Interventions to decrease catheter-related bloodstream infections in the ICU: The Keystone Intensive Care Unit Project. *Am J Infect Control* 36:S171.e1–S171.e5, Dec. 2008.

17. Needleman J., et al.: Nurse-staffing levels and the quality of care in hospitals. *N Engl J Med* 346:1715–1722, May 30, 2002.

18. Aiken L.H., et al.: Effects of hospital care environment on patient mortality and nurse outcomes. *J Nurs Adm* 38:223–229, May 2008.

19. Virtanen M., et al.: Work hours, work stress, and collaboration among ward staff in relation to risk of hospital-associated infection among patients. *Med Care* 47:310–318, Mar. 2009.

Chapter 4

A Risk-Based Approach to Infection Prevention: Creating an Infection Prevention and Control Plan

Barbara Moore Soule, R.N., M.P.A., C.I.C.

Risk is inherent in the delivery of health care services because of the dynamic and complex nature of such services. Vulnerabilities and risks change continually as complex interactions between practitioners, patients, technology, and the environment shift. An infection prevention and control (IPC) program plays a critical role in addressing risk and is thus integral in maintaining a safe work environment and preserving the physical integrity and operations of health care organizations during routine and emergent conditions.

Risks that relate to infection prevention and control can take many forms. Some infection risks are common to many patients or residents (such as device-related infections) or to staff (such as sharps injuries), regardless of the health care setting. Other risks are rare but potentially severe, such as those related to an influx of infectious patients or an emerging infectious disease (such as Sudden Acute Respiratory Syndrome [SARS] or the novel influenza A H1N1 virus, first detected in April 2009). Those risks that are shared among many health care organizations may have similar solutions, but risk-reduction activities must be tailored to the organization to address unique challenges. Risks that seem under control may suddenly change and require new direction for the IPC program. Because of the evolving nature of infection control risks, they must be assessed periodically. Using such a risk-based approach to preventing infections is an ongoing process that forms the cornerstone for an effective IPC program.

USING A RISK-BASED APPROACH TO INFECTION PREVENTION

The Joint Commission's "Infection Prevention and Control" (IC) Standards require that an accredited organization perform an assessment to evaluate infection risks for the organization, establish goals and objectives based on these risks, and develop an IPC plan to guide strategies to achieve the goals and accomplish best outcomes.

Although infection preventionists have long assessed risk—primarily based on populations served, services provided, surveillance data, outbreaks, and gaps in desired practices—the IC standards stipulate that assessing risk and setting goals should be a purposeful and systematic process used to direct a well-designed and thoughtful approach to IPC activities. Several standards form the foundation for this purposeful and systematic process:

- Standard IC.01.03.01, Elements of Performance (EPs) 1 through 5, which delineate the activities for assessing infection risk
- Standard IC.01.04.01, EPs 1 through 5, which describe the development of goals and objectives for the IPC program
- Standard IC.01.05.01, EPs 1 through 3, which provide guidance and the requirements for an IPC program plan

The following sections take a closer look at these standards.

TIP: *The IC standards stipulate that assessing risk and setting goals should be a purposeful and systematic process used to direct a well-designed and thoughtful approach to IPC activities.*

> **STANDARD IC.01.03.01**
>
> The [organization] assesses risks for acquiring and transmitting infections.
>
> **STANDARD IC.01.04.01**
>
> Based on the identified risks, the [organization] sets goals to minimize the possibility of transmitting infections
>
> **STANDARD IC.01.05.01**
>
> The [organization] has an infection prevention and control plan.

EXPLORING IC.01.03.01

The risk assessment process is a thoughtful, systematic examination of infection hazards in the health care environment that could cause harm to patients, staff, families and visitors, or the facility. Standard IC.01.03.01 and its five EPs discuss the types of information an organization must consider when identifying risks for acquiring and transmitting infections.

IC.01.03.01, EP 1: The [organization] identifies risks for acquiring and transmitting infections based on the following: its geographic location, community, and populations served.

The first EP for Standard IC.01.03.01 requires that each organization assess its risk for acquiring and transmitting infection based on its geographic location, the community environment, and the characteristics and behaviors of the populations served.

Infection preventionists can best understand their organization's geographic and community environment by staying in contact with state and local public health services. One way to do this is to register for e-mail alerts sent by the health department to health care providers and organizations, which provide information about community illnesses and trends such as tuberculosis in the homeless population, the occurrence of seasonal influenza, and the incidence of measles, mumps, and other communicable diseases.

The health department also has statistics on population characteristics and health trends that can be helpful when assessing risk. Infection preventionists should develop contacts at their state and local health agencies and, when possible, include them in the risk assessment process.

IC.01.03.01, EP 2: The [organization] identifies risks for acquiring and transmitting infections based on the following: the care, treatment, and services it provides.

Each health care organization provides specific services—such as cardiac care, orthopedic care, pediatric care, long term care, or behavioral health services, just to name a few. The second EP for Standard IC.01.03.01 requires that the risk assessment process include a review of the risks for infection related to the care, treatment, and services the health care organization provides. Some organizations perform highly invasive and risky procedures, such as surgery, interventional radiology, and endoscopy. The infection preventionist in such an organizations should carefully review these procedures to ensure that they are scientifically sound and incorporate current recommendations regarding infection prevention and control. In addition, the infection preventionist must assess whether staff members are following approved infection prevention practices.

A thorough inventory of all services that an organization provides will be invaluable in understanding the risks to patients. For infection preventionists new to an organization, visiting each area of the organization to become familiar with the treatments provided and patients served is worthwhile. The infection preventionist can discuss infection prevention practices with the staff and sometimes may wish to observe those procedures that carry significant risk. For infection preventionists who have worked in an organization for a while, periodically revisiting the departments for this purpose will maintain current knowledge.

IC.01.03.01, EP 3: The [organization] identifies risks for acquiring and transmitting infections based on the following: the analysis of surveillance activities and other infection control data. (*See also* IC.01.02.01, EP 1.)

One of the most valuable sources for quantitative information to guide the risk assessment process is an organization's infection surveillance data. Outcome data on health care–associated infections (HAIs) should be analyzed and used to identify the risk factors related to acquiring and transmitting these infections. Infection preventionists should use surveillance data when conducting a risk assessment and, where possible, compare the organization's data with existing well-validated databases, such as the National Healthcare Safety Network (NHSN).[1]

In addition to outcome data, infection prevention practices should be monitored to identify processes that may prevent or lead to infection. For example, findings from monitoring the following processes can assist in evaluating infection risks:

- Complying with cleaning activities
- Using contact precautions
- Performing hand hygiene
- Using maximal sterile barriers during insertion of central lines
- Keeping the head of the bed elevated for patients with ventilators

The findings of these monitoring efforts may call for improvement in practice or can be used to recognize excellent practice in the organization. Again, comparing organization data with existing well-validated databases can be helpful.

IC.01.03.01, EP 4: The [organization] reviews and identifies its risks at least annually and whenever significant changes occur with input from, at a minimum, infection control personnel, medical staff, nursing, and leadership. (See also IC.03.01.01, EP 1.)

This EP is designed to ensure that infection prevention is attended to by a multidisciplinary group of professionals, each of whom will bring a different perspective to the risk evaluation process. Without input from these personnel, the risk assessment will be incomplete and might miss important considerations.

Those performing a risk assessment should consider new technologies, procedures, medications, vaccines, populations served, services provided, and community characteristics. The assessment should also take into account the requirements of regulatory and accrediting agencies and infection prevention and control guidelines, consensus statements, and guidance documents from groups such as the Centers for Disease Control and Prevention (CDC), the Association for Professionals in Infection Control and Epidemiology (APIC), the Society for Healthcare Epidemiology of America (SHEA), the Infectious Diseases Society of America (IDSA), and others. (See also Chapter 6 for a list of guidance documents.)

This EP also requires an organization to have a continuous relationship with the risk assessment process. The written risk assessment should be a living document that is reviewed and updated at least annually. When there is a change in the organization that could affect infection risk, the assessment must be revisited to determine whether the selected priorities are still appropriate. For example, if an acute care organization acquires a new practice of neurosurgeons that perform high-risk procedures, this should be considered in the risk assessment. Likewise, a significant decrease in nurse–patient staffing ratios may lead to a risk reassessment as these ratios may pertain to increased infection prevention and control risk for patients. Finally, if there is an influx of infectious patients, such as in a community outbreak, the organization's selected risks may need to be reprioritized.

Often, a situation arises in which there is some ambiguity about the risks involved. For example, if clinicians are concerned about whether invasive procedures can be performed at the bedside in a neonatal intensive care unit (NICU) rather than in a distant surgical suite because of the frailty of the neonates, this would be an appropriate time to use the risk assessment process to analyze and specifically assess that issue.

Because of the differences in patient populations, services, the physical environment, and associated infection risks, to comply with this standard an organization must perform a risk assessment for each care setting under its license.

TIP: *The written risk assessment should be a living document that is reviewed and updated at least annually. When there is a change in the organization that could affect infection risk, the assessment must be revisited to determine whether the selected priorities are still appropriate.*

IC.01.03.01, EP 5: The [organization] prioritizes the identified risks for acquiring and transmitting infections. These prioritized risks are documented. (See also IC.01.04.01, EP 1; IC.01.05.01, EP 2; and IC.03.01.01, EP 2.)

Part of the assessment process is to work through and prioritize the identified infection risks of greatest importance and urgency to patients, staff, the patient care environment, and the organization as a whole. Once the analysis is complete, the most significant risks should be selected and documented. This can done be in a stand-alone risk assessment document, but the findings must also be integrated and evident in the IPC plan. The selected risks will be used to develop the goals for the IPC program. (More information about the IPC plan can be found on page 45.) The identified risks will also provide the organization's leadership and the IPC team with information about where to focus infection prevention and control activities.

CRITICAL STEPS IN CONDUCTING A RISK ASSESSMENT

Performing a risk assessment involves a number of steps. (*See* Table 4-1 on page 31.) Some of these steps are introduced in the previous section; the following paragraphs take a closer look at these steps.

Selecting the Appropriate Method and Tools

The risk assessment process begins with the selection of the method and tools that will be used by the organization to assess risk. These are either quantitative or qualitative or a combination of the two.

Using a Quantitative Approach

A typical approach to designing a quantitative risk assessment tool is to create a numeric scoring system based on definitions or criteria. Each risk event is scored with a number. For example, the *probability* of an event occurring could be ranked either on a scale such as "high," "medium," or "low," with corresponding numbers such as 5, 3, or 1, or on a five-point Likert scale that ranks the probability of occurrence from "extremely likely" to "extremely unlikely," with assigned numbers such as 5 (extremely likely) to 1 (extremely unlikely). The *potential severity* of the event then could be ranked from "extremely severe" to "not severe at all," with an assigned number. Depending on the method, numeric values for each variable can be added or multiplied to obtain a total score for each risk event. These scores are ranked and evaluated to select the highest priorities for the IPC program.

For consistent ranking, each category that corresponds to a numeric value must be clearly defined—in other words, what do "high," "medium," and "low" mean? The more precise these definitions, the more consistent and valid the ratings will be when evaluated by different people. Tools 4-1 through 4-7 in the "CD Tools" section, are examples of quantitative risk assessments.

Using a Qualitative Approach

Some organizations prefer to use a qualitative method to assess risk. This involves an inductive approach that begins with the event or process being analyzed and assesses the risk using written descriptions of populations, descriptions of risk, methods of analysis, and outcome indicators.[2] This methodology may incorporate the plans for risk reduction into the actual assessment document or may describe it separately. The qualitative assessment should indicate the priority for each topic, and each priority may be assigned a risk score. (Tools 4-4 and 4-8—both found in the "CD Tools" section—incorporate a qualitative approach into their risk assessments.)

One popular qualitative approach to risk assessment is the gap analysis that uses a priority-setting approach. In this process, the organization asks, "What is the risk at this time?" "Where do we want to be?" or "What is our desired goal?" and "What is the gap?" Each risk is considered and assessed. The final step is to rank each of the items described in the gap analysis to determine the highest priorities. Figure 4-1 on page 33 is an example of a gap analysis for several infection prevention issues.

Another qualitative technique used to evaluate risk is a SWOT (strengths, weaknesses, opportunities, and threats) analysis. For this method, the participants select a particular issue or risk that needs in-depth analysis, such as methicillin-resistant *Staphylococcus aureus* (MRSA) in surgical site infections, and discuss the categories on the SWOT analysis. Once the strengths, weaknesses, opportunities, and threats have been described, the organization can rank the issue or risk based on potential occurrence and severity and can incorporate it into the overall risk assessment (*see* Figure 4-2 on page 34).

Using Criteria to Select a Method

Since there are a number of methods that can be used to assess risk (*see* Sidebar 4-1 on page 35), it is useful to have a set of criteria by which to evaluate the risk assessment method and tools an organization selects. A primary consideration is the comfort of those who will be reviewing the risk assessment and the practicality of the method. If the audience members do not understand the process and tool, they may have a tendency to defer the assessment to others rather

Table 4-1. Steps for Performing an Infection Prevention and Control Risk Assessment

1. Create a Risk Assessment Team or Advisory Group

Form partnerships with
- Key staff (e.g., nursing, medicine, patient safety/quality, pharmacy, laboratory, support services, risk management, employee health, environmental and facility services, others)
- Opinion leaders in the organization
- Administrative and clinical leadership for support and endorsement

2. Establish a Time Line

- Consider strategic planning and budget cycles, as well as committee meetings.
- It should be an annual process, at a minimum.

3. Gather Data and Information

Organizational Data
- Gain access to key reports in the organization needed for the risk assessment, e.g., services provided; populations served, characteristics, and volumes; special environmental issues; microbiological reports and pharmacy antibiotic use data; *See* "Risk Assessment Matrix," Figure 4-1, page 33.
- Review infection prevention and control (IPC) program surveillance data, including multidrug-resistant organism (MDRO) rates and trends.
- Tap into organizational data (medical records, lab records, admission and discharge numbers), as appropriate.
- Review sentinel event reports, risk reports, mortality data, etc.
- Review institutional costs of MDRO infections.

Scientific Data
- Review the literature for new trends—*Journal of the American Medical Association, The New England Journal of Medicine, Clinical Infectious Diseases, Pediatrics, Infection Control and Hospital Epidemiology, American Journal of Infection Control*, and others.
- Link to key Web sites, e.g., those for the Centers for Disease Control and Prevention (CDC), World Health Organization (WHO), Association for Professionals in Infection Control and Epidemiology (APIC), Society for Healthcare Epidemiology of America (SHEA), The Joint Commission, Infectious Diseases Society of America (IDSA), others.

Community Data
- Connect with the local health department to identify trends that may affect MDRO infection risk in the facility.
- Issues of emerging pathogens
- Information concerning special high-risk community populations

4. Develop Systematic Methods and Templates

- Develop a systematic way of collecting and analyzing risk data.
- Turn qualitative data into quantitative information, when possible (*see* "Risk Assessment Matrix," Figure 4-1, page 33).
- Select or design a template.
- Develop a ranking scheme to determine highest priorities.
- Convene a multidisciplinary team in order to rank data to determine priorities.

(continued)

Table 4-1. Steps for Performing an Infection Prevention and Control Risk Assessment (continued)

5. Engage and Educate Others to Assist in Assessment

- Provide support and guidance for others to assess risk related to MDROs.
- Provide educational sessions, as needed, to targeted audiences.
- Share organization's infection control data from surveillance, outbreaks, morbidity, and mortality and highlight incidence and consequences of MDROs.
- Design a simple template for the assessment.

6. Perform the Risk Assessment

- Assemble the team.
- Provide data and information.
- Present the template.
- Complete the template.
- Guide discussion and debate.
- Reach consensus and select highest priorities.
- Present the priorities to the appropriate committee and leadership for support and approval.

7. Use the Priorities to Develop the IPC Program Goals, Objectives, and Activities

- Develop a goal for each selected priority.
- Create an action plan and evaluation process.

8. Disseminate the Information

- Market the risk assessment importance and share results.
- Develop a concise, clear report with key points highlighted.
- Acknowledge those who participate in the process.

This table provides a step-by-step approach to performing an infection prevention and control risk assessment.

Source: Adapted from Arias K.M., Soule B.M. (eds.): *The APIC/JCAHO Infection Control Workbook.* Oakbrook Terrace, IL: Joint Commission Resources, 2005.

---

than be active participants, whereas having a method and tool that is comfortable and easy to use may stimulate involvement. Therefore, it is important to gain approval for both the method and the tool before beginning the process. Some of the criteria for assessing a risk analysis method, system, model, or particular tool include the following[3,4]:

- How appropriate and sound are the underlying methodological assumptions?
- Is the method or tool comprehensive, addressing all necessary information?
- Does the method contain bias? Will the results be accurate and will there be confidence in the results?
- How practical is the method? Is it time-efficient?
- Will those using the process understand it?
- Is there expertise to perform the analysis?
- Is the process fair and ethical?
- Will the results be useful? Will they support the objectives?

Figure 4-1. Sample Gap Analysis for Infection Prevention and Control Risk Assessment

Area/Issue/ Topic/Standard	Current Status	Desired Status	Gap (Describe)	Action Plan and Evaluation	Priority: High, Medium, Low
Incomplete implementation of CDC Hand Hygiene (HH) Guideline (NPSG.01.07.01)	• Guideline approved by ICC • Required elements not implemented throughout the organization	Full implementation of required elements throughout the organization by December 2009, e.g., Category 1A, 1B, 1C	Only 40% of units and services are following CDC HH Guideline and hospital policy.	• Develop proactive implementation plan • Make a leadership priority • Obtain all necessary supplies • Evaluate existing hand hygiene compliance • Provide feedback to staff monthly • Ensure full implementation by December 2009 for all units and services	High
Systematic and proactive surveillance activity to determine usual endemic rates of infections (IC.01.03.01, EP 3)	• Current surveillance is periodic. • Retrospective chart review of a few selected infections • Data not always analyzed in timely manner	• Prospective surveillance for selected infections and populations on an ongoing basis using NHSN methodology	• Lack of IC staff and computer support to perform concurrent and ongoing surveillance • Absence of well designed surveillance plan • Difficult to access laboratory data • Lack of funding for NHSN participation	• Request funding to join NHSN and obtain computer and software to enter and analyze data • Use NHSN methodology and outcomes (infections) monitored by NHSN • Involve ICC in designing surveillance plan priorities • Teach IPC staff about surveillance methodologies • Work with Laboratory Director to design access system for microbiology and other reports • Determine if program exists in 6 months	High
Central line–associated bloodstream infections (CLABSIs) in medical ICU are very high compared to NHSN. (IC.01.03.01, EP 2)	CLABSI in medical ICU at 75th percentile of CDC NHSN benchmark	• Reduce CLABSIs to 25th percentile NHSN benchmark or lower • Strive for zero CLABSIs in MICU for a period of at least 6 months—achieved by Dec 09	• Processes to prevent CLABSIs are not followed consistently among staff. • Supplies not always available • Medical staff do not always adhere to policy.	• Reinforce use of the BSI bundle from IHI • Form team with MICU, IC, MDs, others • Evaluate the bundle processes and the outcomes and report to leadership and ICC monthly	High
Needlesticks in employees increasing (IC.02.03.01)	• The incidence of needlesticks among environmental services (ES) staff is 1%. • Analysis shows that greatest risk is during changing of needle containers.	• Reduce needlesticks in ES staff to equal to or less than 0.2% during next 6 months • Maintain low rate thereafter among all ES staff	• Observations show that needle containers are often overflowing. • There is confusion among nursing and housekeeping staff about responsibility and timing for emptying or changing containers. • Nursing supervisors not aware of issue	• Clarify policy and repeat education to staff about criteria for filling /changing needle containers • Discuss situation with nurse managers—emphasize responsibility • Display ongoing data to show number of weeks without needlesticks • Revaluate needlestick injuries in 3 and 6 months and report to staff and ICC • Evaluate processes implemented for improvement	Medium

This figure shows one way to conduct a gap analysis and assess infection prevention and control risks. CDC, Centers for Disease Control and Prevention; ICC, infection control committee; NHSN, National Healthcare Safety Network; IC, infection control; IPC, infection prevention and control; ICU, intensive care unit; MICU, medical ICU; IHI, Institute for Healthcare Improvement; MD, physician.

To complete the gap analysis, identify the issue and describe the current status, the desired status, and the gap between the two. State the action plan to "close" the gap and evaluation process. Indicate priority among risk issues for the organization.

Source: Barbara M. Soule, R.N., M.P.A., C.I.C.

Figure 4-2. SWOT Analysis: Central Line–Associated Bloodstream Infection Prevention Practices

STRENGTHS	OPPORTUNITIES
• Policy evidence-based and current (see reference) • Current ICU staff competent in approved practices based on periodic assessments • Hand hygiene compliance at 94% and improving • Physician leadership interested in patient safety and improving CLABSI practices	• Education of new staff (nurses and physicians) for all CLABSI practices, e.g., formal education and competency assessments • Identify nurse and physician champions—empower to oversee practices and guide improvements • Revise procedure to assure availability of supplies at all times to enhance compliance, e.g., cart or kit • Use checklist to assure all tasks are carried out; report analysis to staff • Address adherence to MSB with physicians using MD champion • Public reporting of CLABSI rates
WEAKNESSES	THREATS
• Supplies not consistently available in timely manner for insertion procedures • Some physicians do not adhere to MSB • Nonoptimal sites sometimes chosen, e.g., femoral site often selected • Residents do not always feel they are well trained for safe insertion procedures and sites.	• Abuse to nurses who point out lack of adherence to CLABSI insertion protocol • Lack of proper insertion technique and placement in subclavian vein • Interruption of supplies from vendors

This figure shows a SWOT (strengths, weaknesses, opportunities, and threats) analysis related to central line–associated bloodstream infection (CLABSI) prevention practices. ICU, intensive care unit; MSB, maximal sterile barriers; MD, physician.

To perform a SWOT analysis, identify the strengths, weaknesses, opportunities, and threats related to the risk issues being considered. After analysis and discussion, determine numeric rating if using quantitative method or statement of priority if using qualitative method for the risk assessment. It is valuable to perform the SWOT analysis with a team of staff who participate in the process.

Source: Adapted from Marschall J., et al.: Strategies to prevent central line–associated bloodstream infections in acute care hospitals. *Infect Control Hosp Epidemiol* 29(Suppl. 1):S22–S30, 2008.

TIP: *A primary consideration when selecting a risk assessment method is the comfort of those who will be reviewing the assessment and the practicality of the method. If the audience members do not understand the process and tool, they may have a tendency to defer the assessment to others rather than be active participants, whereas a method and tool that is comfortable and easy to use may stimulate involvement.*

Selecting Risk Categories and Topics

Once a method and tools for risk assessment are selected, the next step in the risk assessment process is to designate general risk categories for evaluation. Such categories may include the following:

■ Types of infections, including organisms of epidemiological significance

■ At-risk patient or resident populations

■ Employee risks

- Supplies and equipment risks
- Communication risks
- Emergency preparedness
- Environmental issues
- Geographic considerations
- Community considerations

Once general risk categories are identified, more specific risk events should be identified within each category. For example, in the general category "organisms of epidemiological significance," several multidrug-resistant organisms may be listed, such as MRSA, *Clostridium difficile*, vancomycin-resistant enterococci (VRE), and *Acinetobacter* species. The risks involved with each of these should be evaluated separately. Likewise, under the general category "employee risks," more specific risks may include sharps injuries; exposure to tuberculosis, meningitis, or other infections or influenza; and poor compliance with hand hygiene.

As previously mentioned, risks related to infections can take many forms. They can be viewed as *unexpected* or *involuntary* and include such risks as a community or organizational flood, a bioterrorism event, an influx of a new community population with specific infection risks, or the emergence of a new resistant pathogen. Risks can also be viewed as *expected* or *voluntary*, such as risks involved in the use of central lines to deliver medications or to measure hemodynamics, or the risks involved in the performance of an elective surgical procedure. Both types should be considered for a comprehensive risk assessment. One can also classify risks as *internal* or *external* to the organization. The following sections take a closer look at these two classifications.

External Risks

As the name implies, external risks are risks that come from outside an organization. One type of external risk relates to geographic considerations, such as the climate of different areas. For example, some coastal areas may experience periodic hurricanes or floods and may contend with more waterborne infection risks. Southwestern areas in the United States may experience outbreaks of plague that would be uncommon in other areas of the United States, whereas other geographic areas may have a higher incidence of West Nile virus or hantavirus. As new resistant organisms emerge, they may first show up in one area and move to other states or regions of the country. This occurs globally with influenza viruses and emerging organisms, such as resistant *Klebsiella pneumonia* that produces a broad-spectrum, -lactamase (KPC). Other geographic consid-

---

Sidebar 4-1. Types of Risk Assessment

To help identify infection risk, organizations may use a variety of risk assessment tools. One that is familiar to infection preventionists is the risk assessment that is performed before and during construction or renovation projects. This is generally referred to as the "ICRA" or the proactive risk assessment and is discussed in Chapter 8, page 102.

Another type of assessment is the hazard vulnerability analysis (HVA), which is used to determine the organization's susceptibility to disasters, emergencies, and other untoward events. Some organizations incorporate the infection prevention and control risk assessment into the organization's overall HVA. Results of the HVA allow for the proactive implementation of measures that improve the facility's capability to respond to threats.

When looking at other aspects of infection prevention and control, some organizations adopt the hazard analysis and critical control point (HAACP) assessment used in the food industry.[3] Yet another method used to anticipate and mitigate risk is the failure mode and effects analysis (FMEA), a proactive qualitative and quantitative risk assessment process.[5]

---

erations that can affect local health care facilities include tornadoes, very dry or very moist climates, earthquakes, and volcanic eruptions, all of which may have associated infection risks. Likewise, health care facilities located in strategic urban areas may be more vulnerable to events related to terrorism and may become receiving centers for persons exposed to infectious agents due to a bioterrorism event.

External risks can take other forms. For example, some communities have populations with a high endemic incidence of a particular infection, such as tuberculosis, malaria, HIV/AIDS, or viral hepatitis. Likewise, the socioeconomic level of a population can affect living conditions, which may contribute to poor health practices and the transmission of infections. Families in some areas are less likely than families in other areas to immunize their children against common vaccine-preventable disease. The strength of its public health department influences the community's overall health and infection risks. These factors should be considered as part of the risk assessment process.

Internal Risks

Internal risks—those occurring within an organization—fall into several categories, each with special challenges and characteristics. Risks associated with patients and staff are of primary concern because of these populations' potential exposure to pathogens or injury, with subsequent morbidity and mortality.

An assessment of patient or resident risks will generally be more helpful in guiding IPC activities if it is stratified by subgroups with particular characteristics and behaviors. Such subgroups might include the following:

- Persons who are highly immunocompromised
- Patients in intensive care, behavioral health, long term care, or rehabilitation settings
- Patients undergoing high-risk procedures, such as total joint replacements, cardiovascular surgery, or ventilator-assisted respiratory therapy
- Persons who are very young or old, from premature infants to the frail elderly

Employee-related risks are affected by the general health habits and cultural beliefs of the staff and the staff's awareness of disease transmission. When conducting a risk assessment, it is important to consider staff compliance with infection prevention policies, such as those related to the handling of sharps, use of personal protective equipment (PPE), and performance of appropriate hand hygiene.

In addition, the risk assessment should determine whether effective organizational processes exist for screening and protecting employees, contractual staff, or licensed independent practitioners who may be, or have been, exposed to infectious diseases or who have an infectious or communicable disease. Staff willingness to receive influenza and other vaccinations can determine infection risk for the employees and ultimately the patients or residents. (*See* Chapter 9 for more information on this topic.)

In addition to risks associated with particular populations, certain procedures also present increased risk. Both diagnostic and therapeutic procedures can involve risk for the patient or the care provider. When assessing procedure-related risks, those performing the risk assessment should consider the invasiveness of a procedure, the characteristics of the equipment or devices used in the procedure, the knowledge and technical expertise of those performing the procedure, and how staff adhere to the recommended infection prevention methods. For example, a surgical procedure in which a surgeon performs blind stitching poses a greater sharps-injury risk than a procedure in which visual suturing is performed.

Some noninvasive procedures and treatments that do not appear to have an infection risk have been associated with the transmission of infectious agents. For example, therapeutic modalities that use whirlpools, swimming pools, and other water sources can transmit infection if the equipment is not cleaned and the water is not disinfected regularly.

Infection risks are also present in certain supplies and equipment. For example, reusable supplies and equipment that are moved from patient to patient without being cleaned and disinfected between patient use can transmit pathogenic organisms. An infection preventionist should periodically monitor these practices and consider the results during the risk assessment process.

In addition to the infection risks associated with people and processes of care, the facility itself is vulnerable to or poses risks and hazards, such as the breakdown of utilities during natural or human-caused emergencies, which can result in infection control issues. Likewise, construction and renovation are common in many facilities and pose some danger to immunocompromised and debilitated patients for infection from organisms such as *Aspergillus*. (Further discussion on the environment and its infection control risks can be found in Chapter 8.)

TIP: *Risk assessments generally begin with an analysis of risks that are obvious to the infection prevention and control team and organization leadership. It is important for the team to contemplate events that might occur but that are not fully known or understood, such as an influenza pandemic or an outbreak of an infection of unknown etiology. It is important to review the current literature to learn about new science, studies, and outbreaks that should be considered as potential risks for the organization. The scientific literature and reports from reliable agencies, such as the CDC and state departments of health, can alert organizations to future risk scenarios. (See Table 4-2 on page 37.)*

Table 4-2. Selected Categories and Topics for an Infection Prevention and Control Risk Assessment

Risk Group	Risk Factors
Geographic location	• Natural disasters such as tornadoes, floods, hurricanes, earthquakes • Breakdown of municipal services such as broken water main, strike by sanitation employees • Accidents in the community including mass transit (airplane, train, bus) • Fires involving mass casualties • Intentional acts of: — Bioterrorism — "Dirty bomb" — Contamination of food and water supplies • Prevalence of disease linked with vectors, temperature, other environmental factors
Community	• Community outbreaks of transmissible infectious diseases such as influenza, meningitis • Diseases linked to food and water contamination (such as *Salmonella*, hepatitis A) • Vaccine-preventable illness in unvaccinated populations • Infections associated with primary migrant populations in geographic area • Public health structure • Socioeconomic levels of population • War or displacement
Organization programs and clinical services	• Cardiac service • Orthopedic service • Neonatology • Pediatrics • Dialysis • Long term care • Rehabilitation • Ambulatory clinics • Hospice • Home care • Acute long term care • Behavioral health
Special populations served	• Women and children • Behavioral health patients • Long term care patients • Very young and very elderly • Persons with cognitive and physical deficiencies • Migratory populations • Persons with high-risk-lifestyle issues • Other special needs populations

(continued)

Table 4-2. Selected Categories and Topics for an Infection Prevention and Control Risk Assessment (continued)

Risk Group	Risk Factors
High-risk patients	• Surgical • ICU • NICU • Oncology • Dialysis • Transplant • Patients with MDROs
Health care worker risks	• Understanding disease transmission and prevention • Degree of compliance with infection prevention techniques and policies—hand hygiene, aseptic technique, and use of PPE and isolation • Sharps injuries • Screening for transmissible diseases • Work restriction guidelines • Practice accountability issues
Medical procedures	• Invasiveness of procedure • Equipment used for procedures • Knowledge and technical expertise of those performing procedure • Adequate preparation of patient • Adherence to recommended infection prevention techniques
Equipment and devices	• Cleaning, disinfection, transport, and storage for IV pumps, suction equipment, other equipment • Sterilization or disinfection process for the following: — Scopes — Surgical instruments —Prostheses • Complexity of device (for example, safety needles, robotics) • Skill and experience of user • Safety features: user dependent or automatic • Reuse of single-use devices
Environmental issues	• Construction, renovation, alterations • Notification of construction • ICRAs and construction permits • Utilities performance • Environmental cleaning and disinfection • Adequate environmental staff • Ventilation and utilities • Isolation rooms

(continued)

Table 4-2. Selected Categories and Topics for an Infection Prevention and Control Risk Assessment (continued)

Risk Group	Risk Factors
Emergency preparedness	• Staff education • Managing influx of infectious patients • Triaging patients • Isolation, barriers, PPE • Utilities and supplies • Medications for prophylaxis and treatment • Security • Staff presence during emergencies
Resource limitations	• Nurse staffing • Other clinical and support staffing • Infection preventionist and hospital epidemiologist staffing • Laboratory support services • Environmental services and facilities
Organization's surveillance data	• Catheter-related bloodstream infections • Ventilator-associated pneumonia • Catheter-associated urinary tract infections • Surgical site infections • Gastrointestinal infections • Sepsis • IT support • MDROs
Education and communication	• Education of all staff on infection prevention strategies • Timely education for new diseases or prevention strategies, e.g., MDROs • Communication of infection prevention and control information • Communication of emergency preparedness information • Intra-departmental communication
Supplies and equipment	• Availability of supplies and equipment • Education about appropriate use of supplies • Skill of staff using the equipment • Appropriate cleaning, disinfection, and sterilization • Safe storage

This table suggests categories and specific topics to consider as part of a risk assessment. ICU, intensive care unit; NICU, neonatal ICU; MDRO, multidrug-resistant organisms; PPE, personal protective equipment; IV, intravenous; ICRA, infection control risk assessment; IT, information technology.

Source: Barbara M. Soule, R.N., M.P.A., C.I.C.

Collecting and Using Data for the Assessment

After the risk assessment team determines the general categories and selects the specific risks for evaluation, the team must collect or review data to perform the risk assessment. Many types and sources of data can be helpful, including the following:

- Infection surveillance and employee health data
- Information about the incidence of infections or infection-related deaths in patients or residents
- Findings from cluster or outbreak investigations
- Infection control incident reports
- Equipment failures
- Sharps injuries
- Employee exposures or personal protective device use
- Data from departments such as finance, medical records, and admissions
- Data from local and state health departments

Resources for comparing surveillance data for infections include the NHSN[1] and the Centers for Medicare & Medicaid Services (CMS) Outcome and Assessment Information Set (OASIS)[6] for long term care. Many government agencies mandate the reporting of HAIs that occur in a variety of health care settings, and these data are available in some states for organizational comparisons.

Analyzing Potential Risks

To help analyze potential risks, organizations should ask questions about the risks (*see* Sidebar 4-2, right). One important question is whether a known or potential risk is likely to occur. Another question is how severe the consequences of the risk would be. Yet another important issue to question is whether the organization is adequately prepared to handle the consequences of a potential risk so that any negative effects are eliminated or minimized.

In addition to asking these questions, organizations may wish to consider other factors when analyzing potential risks, such as accreditation and regulatory issues, CMS Conditions of Participation (CoP),[7] and financial impact. Tool 4-1 in the "CD Tools" section, provides an example of a risk analysis that encompasses many of the variables discussed here.

Selecting Priority Infection Risks

Given the limited resources in many IPC programs, addressing every identified risk during a given time period is not always possible. Therefore, using resources wisely by first

---

Sidebar 4-2: Questions for a Risk Assessment

The assessment should address at least two basic questions to analyze risk:

1. What is the probability that a risk event will occur?
2. If it occurs, how severe will it be?

Other questions organizations use to evaluate risk include the following:

- What magnitude of response will be required by the organization?
- How prepared is the organization to respond, should the event occur?
- How will the event affect the target populations (for example, patients, residents, staff)?
- What is the expected frequency of occurrence?
- What is the ability to discover or detect the event?
- What is the leadership support for addressing the event?
- How will the risk affect the financial status of the organization?
- Will the risk affect the physical environment?
- Are there regulations that mandate managing certain risks?
- Will the accreditation status be influenced?

---

addressing those issues that have the most serious potential for harm is imperative. Consequently, after all potential risks are analyzed, the organization must determine which risks should be selected as priorities for the IPC program during a given time period.

When selecting which risks to address, an organization should turn to an organizational risk assessment team, an advisory council, and/or an infection control or patient safety/quality committee to balance data, experience, and information from knowledgeable staff in the organization and to select the risks that pose the greatest potential for morbidity or mortality. Regardless of how the priorities are selected, the organization's leaders should determine approval status and, if approved, provide the needed resources. These approved priorities should then guide the development of goals and measurable objectives for the IPC plan.

Reevaluating the Risk Assessment

Risk identification and assessment are a continuous process. As discussed earlier, the Joint Commission requires, at a minimum, an annual risk assessment. However, it may be prudent and necessary for an organization to examine risks more frequently during the year, if circumstances change. Events such as an outbreak of legionellosis in a hospital or influenza in a nursing home, a new cardiac surgery service, or an outbreak of hepatitis C in an outpatient endoscopy clinic would prompt such a reevaluation.

EXPLORING IC.01.04.01

Once the risk assessment process is complete, writing goals and measurable objectives for the IPC program is essential to formulating the infection prevention plan and determining the activities of the program. As with the risk assessment, engaging the participation of a team of knowledgeable people is the best approach to gaining consensus on how to create goals to address the risk priorities and use them as drivers for key activities.

Standard IC.01.04.01 requires organizations to set goals to minimize the possibility of transmitting infections. The standard and its EPs are discussed in the following sections. Many of the EPs mirror the issues that are considered during risk assessment, demonstrating the link between the two areas.

STANDARD IC.01.04.01

Based on the identified risks, the [organization] sets goals to minimize the possibility of transmitting infections.

IC.01.04.01, EP 1: The [organization's] written infection prevention and control goals include the following: addressing its prioritized risks. (*See also* IC.01.03.01, EP 5; IC.03.01.01, EP 3.)

IC.01.04.01, EP 1, is a clear directive for the IPC team to use the risk assessment results to develop the goals for the IPC program. The goals should be directly linked to the highest priorities to show a continuous process from analysis to action. For example, if the incidence of VRE is identified as a significant risk for the organization, there should be a goal to reduce the incidence. The IPC plan will probably include other goals for maintaining the program that are not ranked as high priorities in the analysis but that are necessary for programmatic success.

Each goal should be accompanied by a measureable objective, an action plan, and an evaluation process to determine whether the objective has been met. A discussion of writing goals and objectives is found in Sidebar 4-3 on page 42.

IC.01.04.01, EP 2: The [organization's] written infection prevention and control goals include the following: limiting unprotected exposure to pathogens. (*See also* IC.02.01.01, EPs 2 and 3; IC.03.01.01, EP 3.)

IC.01.04.01, EP 2, refers to the measures that an organization uses to protect patients, residents, staff, visitors, and others from contact with potentially infectious organisms. The use of aseptic technique, hand hygiene, and PPE (such as gowns, gloves, masks, and respirators) falls into this category. Isolation procedures, engineering controls for airborne pathogens, barriers during construction, and safety hoods in the laboratory would be appropriate topics or issues to consider under this goal as well. (Many of these strategies are discussed in detail in Chapter 6.)

IC.01.04.01, EP 3: The [organization's]s written infection prevention and control goals include the following: limiting the transmission of infections associated with procedures. (*See also* IC.03.01.01, EP 3.)

Patients are exposed to many procedures that are designed to diagnose, improve, or maintain health. As previously mentioned, some of these procedures carry significant risk for infection because they are invasive or complex in nature (for example, surgical procedures). The health status of the patient, the duration of the procedure, and the state of the wound (for example, clean or dirty) all influence whether a person may experience a postoperative surgical site infection (SSI). For example, healthy patients having clean hernia repairs have a relatively low risk for SSI, whereas those having bowel surgery after trauma have a higher risk.

Because of the risks for infection associated with surgery, each area of care in the surgical services, including preoperative, perioperative, and postoperative settings, should have goals and related policies and procedures to assure minimal infection risk to patients. Settings where invasive procedures are performed require constant vigilance from the IPC team to ensure that effective infection prevention policies and practices are in place. These settings can include, but are not limited to, the following:

■ Interventional radiology

- Endoscopy and bronchoscopy settings
- Injection clinics
- Anesthesia

IC.01.04.01, EP 4: The [organization's] written infection prevention and control goals include the following: limiting the transmission of infections associated with the use of medical equipment, devices, and supplies. (*See also* IC.02.02.01, EPs 1–5; IC.03.01.01, EP 3.)

The IPC program is responsible for overseeing the processes that ensure safe use of medical devices—such as intravenous (IV) needles and tubing, bronchoscopes, and ventilators—and the appropriate management of equipment and sterile supplies. As such, the goals and associated policies and procedures related to cleanliness, disinfection, sterilization, storage, and transport of equipment, sterile supplies, and single-use devices should be reviewed and approved by the IPC oversight body. Compliance with infection prevention practices should be monitored as delegated by the organization (*see* Chapter 6 for more information).

IC.01.04.01, EP 5: The [organization's] written infection prevention and control goals include the following: improving compliance with hand hygiene guidelines. (*See also* IC.03.01.01, EP 3; NPSG.07.01.01, EP 1.)

Hand hygiene is addressed in National Patient Safety Goal NPSG.07.01.01, and compliance is required for *all* accredited organizations. Goals and objectives related to hand hygiene can include a specified target for hand hygiene compliance, improved hand hygiene technique, and improved accessibility of hand hygiene products. Chapter 11 of this publication describes strategies for meeting this goal. In addition, recommendations for monitoring hand hygiene are available in the monograph *Measuring Hand Hygiene Adherence: Overcoming the Challenges* published by the Joint Commission.[8]

EXPLORING IC.01.05.01

When the risk assessment is completed, priorities are selected, and goals and objectives are established, the infection prevention and control team can finalize its infection prevention and control plan. Like the IPC program, the IPC plan must be dynamic and designed to respond quickly to changes and demands in the health care environment. These changes may be related to issues such as emerging infectious diseases, new

Sidebar 4-3: Writing Clear Goals and Measurable Objectives

Infection prevention and control (IPC) goals are general statements that establish intent, direction, and broad parameters for the desired achievements of an IPC program. For example, a goal might state the following:

> The IPC program will reduce central line–associated bloodstream infections (CLABSIs) in the intensive care unit (ICU).

This statement clearly communicates intent, but because no specific numeric target or date exists, one cannot determine by what amount the CLABSIs in the ICU will be reduced or the time line for achieving this outcome.

Objectives of the IPC program are statements of specific intent or desired achievements for the program. Objectives should state what will be achieved (in numeric values, when possible), provide a specific time frame when the action will be completed, and identify the population, location, or process being targeted. A written objective should be measurable. An objective for the previously stated goal could be stated as follows:

> The medical ICU will have zero CLABSIs for a period of at least three months by December 2010.

Another objective might be as follows:

> Reduce CLABSIs from the 75th percentile to below the 25th percentile of the National Healthcare Safety Network (NHSN) comparable data in the medical ICU by June 2010.

Goals and measurable objectives establish targets for performance improvement activities and allow the IPC program to evaluate progress and success or failure in these efforts. (*See* Table 4-3 on page 43.) After goals and objectives have been established, they should be used to develop the IPC plan.

Source: Adapted from Schreck M., Watson S.: Education and training. In Carrico R. (ed.): *The APIC Text of Infection Control and Epidemiology*, 3rd ed. Washington DC: Association for Professionals in Infection Control and Epidemiology, 2009, pp. 11-1–11-10.

Table 4-3. Sample Goals and Objectives for the Infection Prevention and Control Program

Goal	Examples of Measurable Objectives
Reduce ventilator-associated pneumonias (VAP) in the intensive care unit (ICU)	• Reduce VAP by equal to or greater than 50%, from 1.4/1,000 ventilator days to 0.7/1,000 ventilator days in the medical ICU (MICU), by June 2009 • Achieve zero VAPs for minimum of 3 months by January 2010 in the MICU • Assess daily whether the need for a ventilator's documented for 98% of ICU ventilated patients by January 2010
Decrease sharps injuries in employees	• Reduce needlestick injuries among direct care and support staff by at least 60% from the 2008 rate within first six months of 2009 • Reduce scalpel injuries in surgical staff by 80% from current rate with implementation of "pass zone" by July 2009
Increase immunizations in the organization	• Identify and immunize at least 90% of eligible patients with pneumococcal vaccine by December 2009 • Immunize 100% eligible staff in organization with influenza vaccine within 6 months of initiating a mandatory flu vaccine program
Increase hand hygiene compliance	• Achieve at least 95% compliance with hand hygiene policy on at least 80% of nursing units by October 2009
Prevent transmission of infectious diseases in the organization	• Achieve at least 98% compliance with contact isolation policy for patients with methicillin-resistant *Staphylococcus aureus* (MRSA) and *Clostridium difficile* on all patient care units during 2010
Maintain consistent cleaning of reusable patient equipment in the ICUs	• Achieve at least 98% compliance with appropriate cleaning procedures for reusable direct care patient equipment during patient stay and at discharge in the MICU, surgical ICU, and neonatal ICU during 2010
Infection prevention and control staff notify staff about construction, renovation, or alteration in facility before beginning work	• Achieve equal to or greater than 95% notification to infection prevention and control staff before any construction, renovation, or alteration occurs in facility for all appropriate (per policy) construction projects by October 2009
Prepare for the response to an influx or risk of influx of infectious patients	• Meet equal to or greater than 90% of Hospital Emergency Incident Command System (HEICS) plan requirements related to infectious patients during at least three drills in 2010

This table provides examples of goals and objectives that can be used in an infection prevention and control (IPC) program.

Source: Barbara M. Soule, R.N., M.P.A., C.I.C.

requirements for mandatory reporting of HAI information, an organization's acquisition of new services, or major construction projects.

The IPC plan should be a succinct, useful document that identifies priorities and needs, sets goals and objectives, lists strategies to meet the goals, and includes the evaluation process. The plan may include or append narratives, policies and procedures, protocols, practice guidelines, clinical paths, care maps, or other helpful documents. The process of creating the IPC plan is covered in Standard IC.01.05.01, which is discussed in the following sections.

STANDARD IC.01.05.01

The [organization] has an infection prevention and control plan.

TIP: *The IPC plan should be a succinct, useful document that identifies priorities and needs, sets goals and objectives, lists strategies to meet the goals, and includes the evaluation process.*

IC.01.05.01, EP 1: When developing infection prevention and control activities, the [organization] uses evidence-based national guidelines or, in the absence of such guidelines, expert consensus. (*See also* IC.01.02.01, EP 1.)

IC.01.05.01, EP 1, is intended to ensure that an organization continually updates its IPC program and plan and that they are based on the best scientific evidence or expert consensus to guide decisions about patient care, maintenance of the environment, staff safety, and other elements of the program. As previously mentioned, many guidelines and guidance documents are available to help organizations in this effort. The infection prevention and control team should refer to these references when developing and evaluating the plan.

IC.01.05.01, EP 2: The [organization's] infection prevention and control plan includes a written description of the activities, including surveillance, to minimize, reduce, or eliminate the risk of infection. (*See also* IC.01.02.01, EPs 1–3; IC.01.03.01, EP 5; IC.02.01.01, EP 1; IC.03.01.01, EP 4.)

The IPC plan is most helpful to staff if the activities are clearly stated in writing. Although the Joint Commission does not require all programs specifically to have a written IPC plan, documenting the activities eliminates ambiguity as to how the program's resources will be allocated and used and also helps to maintain focus. The plan should be written in a simple style and be easily understandable and accessible to the infection prevention and control team and other staff who participate in the activities.

Key components of the IPC plan are the scope and methods for surveillance, which differ depending on the setting and populations served. Each organization must design a surveillance program based on its characteristics, populations, services, risks, and requirements. (*See* Sidebar 4-5 on page 47.) Although there is no nationally standardized method for identifying, collecting, managing, analyzing, and reporting data on infections, the CDC's NHSN surveillance methodology and criteria are increasingly being used by a variety of health care organizations and settings worldwide.[1] Surveillance definitions have been established for hospital,[1] dialysis unit,[1] long term care,[9] and home health care and home hospice[10] settings.

In many ambulatory care settings, surveillance is focused primarily on processes or practices—such as the percentage of eligible patients who receive immunizations, compliance rates for hand hygiene, and assessment of environmental cleanliness—rather than on outcomes of care, such as infections. However, ambulatory settings performing invasive procedures can measure infections, including those related to endoscopy or surgical procedures.

IC.01.05.01, EP 3: The [organization's] infection prevention and control plan includes a written description of the process to evaluate the infection prevention and control plan. (*See also* IC.03.01.01, EP 1.)

In IC.01.05.01, EP 3, the Joint Commission has included the requirement to delineate how the IPC program's goals and objectives will be evaluated. The advantage of designing this into the plan is to create a mechanism that will guide the evaluation process and promote periodic reevaluation. This helps ensure that the infection control committee, patient safety committee, and organization leadership agree on the evaluation process and can align it with organizational performance evaluation methods. Strategies for evaluating the IPC program are discussed in Chapter 10.

DEVELOPING AN INFECTION PREVENTION AND CONTROL PLAN

To develop an IPC plan, staff should consider convening a group that will work collaboratively to contribute various perspectives and expertise to the process. Issues that should be addressed in the development process include the following:

- Effective management of the IPC program
- Infection risks and prevention and control strategies
- The evaluation process
- Occupational health
- Emergency planning
- Communication
- Applicable requirements of government, accrediting, and other organizations
- Leadership support and resources allocated

An IPC plan can consist of several sections. One section may be general background information that delineates the scope of the program and that might include the mission of the organization and how the IPC program supports the mission. This section may also discuss the organization's size and type, geographic location, populations served, reporting structure, statement of authority, and hours of operation. It may also describe the coverage and services offered by the infection prevention and control team, such as consultation, education, product evaluation, and collection and analysis of surveillance data and information. This section can include how the IPC program and staff participate in patient safety and performance improvement and the sentinel event process and other activities.

The general background section of the IPC plan, although reviewed annually and updated as necessary, probably will change little from year to year unless there are major shifts in the program.

Another key section of the IPC plan is the statement of the risk priorities, goals, objectives, action plans, and evaluation methods for a given time period, such as a year. This section would evolve from the risk assessment process and is likely to be updated after each risk assessment. Examples of infection prevention and control plans that incorporate risk assessment results are found in the "CD Tools" section.

An organization may wish to include a third section of the IPC plan that consists of support documents, such as care plans, decision algorithms, clinical pathways, or key procedures. The surveillance plan and the process for outbreak investigation may also be integrated into the overall IPC plan, or they can stand as separate written documents.

Regardless of how an organization chooses to design its infection prevention and control plan, it should be a useful document. Table 4-4 on page 46 provides suggestions for content for an IPC program plan. Some tips for writing an infection prevention and control plan are shown in Sidebar 4-4, below.

Sidebar 4-4: Tips for Writing an Infection Prevention and Control Plan

- Develop an outline and create a table of contents for the written infection prevention and control (IPC) plan.
- Identify the local, state, and federal regulations and other requirements (that is, accreditation standards and infection prevention and control standards and guidelines) that are applicable to the specific heath care setting.
- Perform a risk assessment.
- Establish and prioritize goals and develop measurable objectives.
- Develop strategies to meet the IPC program's goals and objectives.
- Establish mechanisms for evaluating the effectiveness of the IPC program.
- Set up a system to be notified of any new services or procedures.
- Develop a time line and assign responsibility for periodically reviewing the plan.
- Ask for review and comments from key personnel and revise, as needed.
- Network with infection preventionists who practice in similar health care settings to obtain and share information needed to develop and maintain the IPC program.

Table 4-4. Suggested Content for an Infection Prevention and Control (IPC) Program Plan

Background information	• Information about the organization • Mission/vision/structure/processes of the IPC program • Scope of services • Staffing and credentials • Decision authority for IPC program (authority statement) • Integration of IPC program with patient safety and performance improvement • Committee functions and responsibilities • Education of staff, patients, and infection prevention and control team • Consultation services • Role in emergency preparedness and management • Public health partnerships • Relationships with occupational health/employee health • Regulatory compliance • Specific patient care or environmental issues • Other special issues
Action plan	• Risk assessment priorities • Goals and objectives • Action plans • Evaluation methods • Responsible persons
Supportive documents	• Surveillance plan • Outbreak investigation • Education plan • Key procedures and policies • Care plans • Decision algorithms
Other	• Research activities • Performance improvement activities • Key resources • Budget

This table offers some content suggestions an organization should consider when developing an IPC plan.

Source: Barbara M. Soule, R.N., M.P.A., C.I.C.

Sidebar 4-5. Infection Prevention and Control Plans for Non–Acute Health Care Settings

Much of health care is provided outside the traditional acute care setting. Ambulatory care services are provided in ambulatory surgical centers, physicians' offices, dialysis centers, clinics, and imaging centers. Home care is provided in a patient's home by caregivers who have variable skill levels. Long term care settings may provide skilled nursing, rehabilitation, or acute care. Behavioral health care is delivered in diverse settings, such as residential facilities, private practices, community centers, drug rehabilitation centers, special hospital units, and jails and prisons. Each of these diverse health care settings has unique challenges for planning and implementing an infection prevention and control (IPC) program.

Regardless of the health care setting, the principles of infection transmission, prevention, and control are the same. Some, but not all, guidelines, standards, and position statements for hospitals can be adapted to other health care settings. Therefore, the risk assessment and the design and scope of the IPC program must be based on risks in each setting. If a health care system encompasses more than one type of health care setting, the IPC plan can be a separate document for each setting, they can be combined into one document for all settings, provided that there is a clear delineation of the needs and plans for each setting, each patient population, and the services provided.

SUMMARY

This chapter has described the following three key components of the IPC program related to best practices and the Joint Commission "Infection Prevention and Control" standards:
- The infection risk assessment
- The process of developing goals and objectives based on the identified risks and organizational and programmatic considerations
- The infection prevention and control plan

Together, these components form the foundation for the IPC program. Careful and thorough preparation in these areas by an organization's infection prevention and control team and key staff will result in a program that can effectively prevent infections and improve patient safety.

FURTHER RESOURCES

Refer to the following tools and resources for helpful examples of how to perform an infection control risk assessment, write goals and objectives, and develop an infection prevention and control plan.

CD Tools

Tool 4-1: SkyRidge Medical Center Infection Control Risk Analysis

Tool 4-2: Cape Cod Healthcare—Infection Control Risk Analysis Sample Risk Assessment Grid and Instructions

Tool 4-3: Luke Hospital—Infection Control Risk Assessment Hazard Scoring Matrix Gap Analysis

Tool 4-4: Riverview Medical Center Infection Prevention Risk Assessment

Tool 4-5: Instructions to Infection Control Committee Regarding Risk Assessment

Tool 4-6: Sample Quantitative Risk Assessment Grid

Tool 4-7: Johnson City Medical Center Risk Assessment and IC Plan

Tool 4-8: Mayo Clinic Risk Assessment and IC Plan

Tool 4-9: Meriter Hospital Infection Prevention and Control Plan

Tool 4-10: SkyRidge Medical Center Infection Control Program Plan

Web Site
- Society for Risk Analysis: http://www.sra.org

Additional Readings

- Centers for Disease Control and Prevention: *Focus on Prevention: Conducting a Hazard Risk Assessment.* http://www.cdc.gov/niosh/docs/2003-139/2003-139.html.

- Forrest S.: Risk assessment matrix for MRSA. *Nurs Times* 96:38–39, 2007.

- Gibson L.L., Rose J.B., Haas C.H.: Use of quantitative microbial risk assessment for evaluation of the benefits of laundry sanitation. *Am J Infect Control* 27:S34–S39, Dec. 1999.

- Gustafson T.L.: Practical risk-adjusted quality control charts for infection control. *Am J Infect* 28:406–414, Dec. 2000.

- Health and Safety Executive 2006: *Five Steps to Risk Assessment.* http://www.hse.gov.uk/workplacetransport/information/riskassessment.htm.

- Jenkins, B.D.: *Risk Analysis, Risk Assessment, Risk Management,* 1998. http://www.nr.no/~abie/RiskAnalysis.htm.

- Joint Commission Resources: Assessing and addressing infection control risks: How does your organization measure up? Part 1. *The Source* 4:1–5, Sep. 2006.

- Joint Commission Resources: Assessing and addressing infection control risks: How does your organization measure up? Part 2 *The Source* 4:1–5, Oct. 2006.

- Marx D.A., Slonim A.D.: Assessing patient safety risk before the injury occurs: An introduction to sociotechnical probabilistic risk modeling in health care. *Qual Saf Health Care* 13:33–38, Dec. 2003.

REFERENCES

1. Centers for Disease Control and Prevention: *National Healthcare Safety Network (NHSN).* http://www.cdc.gov/nhsn/index.html (accessed Jun. 2, 2009).

2. Robertson C., O'Boyle C., Connor S.B.: Methods of analysis. In Carrico R. (ed.): *The APIC Text of Infection Control and Epidemiology,* 3rd ed. Washington, DC: Association for Professionals in Infection Control and Epidemiology, 2009, pp. 30-1–30-8.

3. Larson E., Aiello A.E.: Systematic risk assessment methods for the infection control professional. *Am J Infect Control* 34:323–326, 2006.

4. Corvello V., Merkhoffer M.: *Risk Assessment Methods: Approaches for Assessing Health and Environmental Risks.* New York: Plenum Press, 1993.

5. Joint Commission on Accreditation of Healthcare Organization: *Failure Mode and Effects Analysis: Proactive Risk Reduction,* 2nd ed. Oakbrook Terrace, IL: Joint Commission Resources, 2005.

6. Centers for Medicare & Medicaid Services (CMS): §484.20 Condition of Participation: Reporting OASIS information. In *State Operations Manual: Appendix B—Guidance to Surveyors: Home Health Agencies.* http://www.cms.hhs.gov/manuals/downloads/som107ap_b_hha.pdf (accessed Jun. 2009).

7. Centers for Medicare & Medicaid Services (CMS): §482.42 Condition of Participation: Infection Control. In *State Operations Manual: Appendix A—Survey Protocol, Regulations and Interpretive Guidelines for Hospitals.* http://www.cms.hhs.gov/manuals/downloads/som107ap_a_hospitals.pdf (accessed Jul. 2009).

8. The Joint Commission: *Measuring Hand Hygiene Adherence: Overcoming the Challenges.* http://www.jointcommission.org/NR/rdonlyres/68B9CB2F-789F-49DB-9E3F-2FB387666BCC/0/hh_monograph.pdf (accessed Jun. 2009).

9. McGeer A., et al.: Definitions of infection for surveillance in long-term care facilities. *Am J Infect Control* 19:1–7, Feb. 1991.

10. Embry F.C., Chinnes L.F.: *APIC-HICPAC Surveillance Definitions for Home Health Care and Home Hospice Infections,* Feb. 2008. http://www.apic.org/AM/Template.cfm?Section=Definitions_and_Surveillance&Template=/CM/ContentDisplay.cfm&ContentFileID=9898 (accessed Apr. 2009).

Chapter 5

Planning for and Managing Infectious Disease Emergencies

Ruth M. Carrico, Ph.D., R.N., C.I.C.; and Terri Rebmann, Ph.D., R.N., C.I.C.

The spread of the novel H1N1 influenza A virus that swept Mexico and infiltrated almost every other country around the world in 2009 refocuses the attention of the health care community on the risk and probability of an infectious disease emergency. The Joint Commission requires organizations to plan how they will respond to an infectious disease emergency and use a multidisciplinary, interactive approach to such a situation.

In the "Infection Prevention and Control" (IC) standards, the concept of responding to an infectious disease emergency is addressed in Standard IC.01.06.01. This chapter takes a close look at this standard and discusses how organizations can adequately comply with its requirements.

STANDARD IC.01.06.01

The organization prepares to respond to an influx of potentially infectious patients.

PLANNING FOR AN INFLUX OF INFECTIOUS PATIENTS

An organization's ability to deliver care, treatment, and services is threatened when the organization is ill prepared to respond to a real or potential epidemic or infections likely to require expanded or extended care capabilities over a prolonged period. Therefore, it is important for an organization to plan how to prevent the introduction of the infection into the organization, how to quickly recognize that existing patients have become infected, and/or how to contain the risk or spread of the infection.

Standard IC.01.06.01 requires that an organization—through its individual leadership structure—have a thorough knowledge of existing capabilities for responding to an influx of

infectious patients and be able to evaluate those capabilities in relation to anticipated needs and identified weaknesses. The activities and plans used by the infection prevention and control function must continue to be dynamic, visible, and comprehensive. This standard aims to promote the type and intensity of planning that will result in improved and thoughtful care during times that challenge the entire organization.

An organization's planned response to an infectious disease emergency should have a basis in competent infection prevention practices and should build on the prevention practices and processes included in everyday best practices. The planned response may include a broad range of options, including the following:

- Temporary halting of services and/or admissions
- Delay of transfers or discharges
- Limitation of visitors within an organization
- Full activation of the organization's emergency management plan

The actual response depends on issues such as the extent to which the community is affected by the epidemic or infection, the types of services the organization offers, and the organization's capabilities.

TIP: *An organization's ability to deliver care, treatment, and services is threatened when the organization is ill prepared to respond to a real or potential epidemic or infections likely to require expanded or extended care capabilities over a prolonged period. Therefore, it is important for an organization to plan how to prevent the introduction of the infection into the organization, how to quickly recognize that existing patients have become infected, and/or how to contain the risk or spread of the infection.*

The underpinning of a comprehensive planning process must include several important factors:

1. The health care organizations in a given community represent an important part of the essential infrastructure of that community. Maintenance of a health care process provides an important social strength. Loss of adequate health care has a severe destabilizing impact on a community.

2. Preplanning is essential if an organization is to remain agile in its ability to carry out its missions during challenging situations.

3. The planning process includes the identification and development of strategies that prevent the introduction of infection, recognize such situations, and promote activities and systems that are capable of containing the infectious events.

4. Vital to the understanding of this standard is that the response of an individual organization depends on a variety of factors. As previously mentioned, these include the impact of the event on the community, the types of services offered by the organization, and the individual organization's capabilities. Developing response plans requires that an organization be realistic in assessing its capabilities and challenge itself as it conducts preparatory efforts. As discussed in Chapter 4, performing a risk assessment for vulnerabilities related to infectious disease emergencies will assist organizations in customizing their plans based on unique characteristics, such as geographic setting, community resources, populations served, and ability to receive supplies during a crisis.

5. The ability of an organization to respond is directly related to the ability of its health care workforce to competently apply infection prevention activities during routine job performance, so those skills must be hardwired into the process of care within the health care facility.

Looking at the Broader Picture

Standard IC.01.06.01 clearly implies the need to plan, communicate, and interact with external partners beyond the historic collaboration with the U.S. public health service. In addition to planning on a small scale, organizations must also plan for emergencies on a larger scale. Recognizing that many staff move from facility to facility, promoting harmony among plans increases the ability of staff to effectively adhere

to the plan. Working with the facility emergency manager, local emergency management agency (EMA), local hospital association, and other area health care organizations will help promote this harmony among responders and can form a basis for long-term collaboration.

TIP: *The health care organizations in a given community represent an important part of the essential infrastructure of that community. Maintenance of a health care process provides an important social strength. Loss of adequate health care has a severe destabilizing impact on a community.*

EXPLORING IC.01.06.01

Like all other standards, IC.01.06.01 has several elements of performance (EPs) that outline how an organization can comply with the standard. For this standard, there are six basic EPs. The following sections examine these EPs and provide tips and strategies on how to comply.

IC.01.06.01, EP 1: The [organization] identifies resources that can provide information about infections that could cause an influx of potentially infectious patients. These resources may include local, state, and federal public health systems.

To comply with IC.01.06.01, EP 1, organizations may want to consider creating trending reports of significant microbiologic organisms identified in patients within the organization, reviewing antibiograms, accessing reportable disease summaries from the state and local health departments, reviewing information and investigations performed by the Centers for Disease Control and Prevention (CDC), and incorporating all this information into the organization's risk assessment. (*See* Chapter 4.)

IC.01.06.01, EP 2: The [organization] obtains current clinical and epidemiological information from its resources regarding new infections that could cause an influx of potentially infectious patients.

Examples of how IC.01.06.01, EP 2 can be met may include items such as evidence of communication regarding trends seen in the community and other health care facilities, knowledge of relevant core performance measure results (for example, community-acquired pneumonia and its etiology), and identification of emerging infections or changes in susceptibilities of organisms identified through review of antimicrobial utilization or communication with clinical pharmacists.

IC.01.06.01, EP 3: The [organization] has a method for communicating critical information to licensed independent practitioners and staff about emerging infections that could cause an influx of potentially infectious patients.

Examples of activities that demonstrate how IC.01.06.01, EP 3, could be met include newsletters, e-mails, Webcasts, and other types of communication with the medical staff, schools of nursing and allied health, and residents. Information in such communication could relate to changes in patient presentation or clinical course when an infectious agent or process is identified. Methods of communication should enable communication to occur before, during, and after an influx of patients.

IC.01.06.01, EP 4: The [organization] describes, in writing, how it will respond to an influx of potentially infectious patients. One acceptable response is to decide not to accept patients.

Written policies and procedures, program plans, training courses, checklists, and signage are examples of how IC.01.06.01, EP 4 may be met. Evidence of communication regarding these policies, procedures, and plans should be available for review and reference.

IC.01.06.01, EP 5: If the [organization] decides to accept an influx of potentially infectious patients, then the [organization] describes in writing its methods for managing these patients over an extended period of time.

Written policies, procedures, and plans should be in place and demonstrate the multidisciplinary scope and involvement necessary to manage patients over an extended period of time. There should be evidence of communication and work with the organization's emergency management function. There should also be evidence of staff training and education regarding these activities.

IC.01.06.01, EP 6: When the [organization] determines it is necessary, the [organization] activates its response to an influx of potentially infectious patients.

To meet IC.01.06.01, EP 6, organizations should have knowledge of the process for initiating or activating the organization's response. The infection preventionist should be aware of his or her role in the process.

ADDRESSING THE CORNERSTONES OF PREPAREDNESS

Emergency management planning—particularly planning for emergencies that involve infectious disease—is never finished; it is an ongoing process that evolves as threats change and gaps in planning are identified. In this way, emergency planning is aligned with continuous process evaluation and improvement and is part of a state of readiness. An effective emergency preparedness program incorporates continuous process evaluation and improvement into all aspects of the program and provides a mechanism for evaluation and improvement.

Through its EPs, Standard IC.01.06.01 addresses the cornerstones of an effective emergency preparedness program. These cornerstones include recognition, response, containment, and communication. Although distinct, the cornerstones are part of a continuous and interconnected process and must be viewed as cyclical and not linear. (Figure 5-1 on page 52 demonstrates this cyclical process.) The following sections examine these cornerstones more closely.

Recognition

Recognition provides the organization with the ability to contain an infectious patient prior to disease transmission to other patients, staff, and the community. It is doubtful that many organizations could identify the first in a group or cluster of infectious patients, but the goal should be to have regular care practices in place that serve to recognize key indicators or symptoms, minimize transmission, and initiate response as early as possible. Recognition could involve identification of patients presenting with specific types of signs, symptoms, or complaints. Once staff recognize these patients, response or containment activities can begin. Therefore, care processes and systems that incorporate safety measures can be a great asset in early recognition.

Practices implemented in one hospital demonstrate this type of approach. University Hospital is a 404-bed level 1 trauma center with large oncology and women's health services in the mideast area of the United States. In addition, an active infectious diseases service operates the largest comprehensive

Figure 5-1. Cornerstone Elements in a Continuous Emergency Preparedness Program

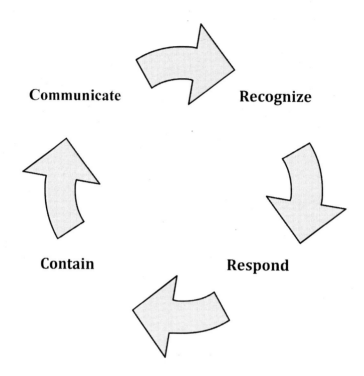

This figure illustrates the continuous nature of the emergency preparedness process.

Source: Ruth M. Carrico, Ph.D., R.N., C.I.C.

HIV/AIDS clinic in the region. In the early 1990s, the hospital employee health department noted a subtle increase in tuberculosis (TB) skin test conversions among staff. Investigation revealed that there had been several cases of active TB that had been delayed in diagnosis. The most common reason for the delay was that patients presented with symptoms consistent with community-acquired pneumonia (CAP), and although TB infection was on the differential diagnosis, it was not a primary consideration, and preventive strategies were not immediately initiated. Diagnostic testing was performed on day 2 or 3 of hospitalization. These delays represented workplace exposures for health care personnel.

In response to an investigation, a systems change was initiated. This change recognized the changing populations and the increased risks for health care personnel. A protocol was developed so that all patients admitted with CAP were immediately placed in airborne infection isolation until TB was ruled out. This systems change resulted in a process that supported rapid evaluation so isolation could be quickly discontinued once a transmissible cause was ruled out.

Over the course of the next 10 years, patients with unsuspected TB were isolated through this early risk identification process. The systems approach supported this preventive activity, and the safety of the care environment has been a positive outcome.

Interestingly, this approach has also resulted in the isolation of patients with pneumonia as a result of influenza, supporting an improved safety environment for patients, staff, and families. Staff are also well versed in obtaining optimal respiratory specimens for laboratory testing and doing so in a safe manner. In addition, this process has underscored the risks of respiratory infection transmission with staff and the potential relationships between patient illness and staff illness. Each organization needs to evaluate its unique risks and implement programs that address them. This program may not be suitable for all facilities, but it demonstrates the conceptual basis for the approach.

Response

The example from University Hospital demonstrates the utility of an early recognition and early risk identification processes. These enable early implementation of a response process. Once a risk has been identified, appropriate response activities can begin. Emergency preparedness efforts work for early recognition so response begins earlier in the continuum.

Response includes mechanisms that contain the infectious patient. Examples may include the use of isolation and/or quarantine. It is important to clearly distinguish between these two terms:

- *Isolation* is the separation and confinement of individuals known to be or suspected of being (based on signs, symptoms, or laboratory findings) infected with a contagious disease to prevent them from transmitting the disease to others.
- *Quarantine* is the compulsory physical separation, including restriction of movement, of populations or groups of healthy individuals who have potentially been exposed to a contagious disease.

Additional information regarding isolation and quarantine can be found on the CDC's Emergency Preparedness and Response Web site, at http://emergency.cdc.gov/preparedness/quarantine.

Response efforts may also include implementing an incident management system, as needed. Implementing an incident management system requires that there be an ability to identify responsible individuals or functions on a 24-hours-a-day, 7-days-a-week, 365-days-a-year basis.

Containment

Once a situation involving a known or suspected infectious patient(s) has been identified, containment becomes a primary initiative. This can be accomplished through actions such as isolation or segregation, use of protective equipment by the health care worker, masking the patient if his or her condition allows, cohorting with other patients with the shared diagnosis, or combinations of these actions. Each individual situation will need to be evaluated and containment activities that are specific to the cause or suspected cause of the infection, modes of transmission, and individuals involved will need to be implemented. (*See* Figure 5-2 on page 54 for an algorithm organizations can use to help manage and place patients who require airborne precautions.)

Containment might also require drastic measures such as increasing surge capacities beyond existing capabilities. This may include allocating physical space for patients or altering the care environment, such as increasing negative pressure surge capacity environments that allow for airborne infection isolation. The complexities involved in this process underscore the need for preplanning. (*See* Sidebar 5-1 on page 55 for a tool that may be helpful in planning for containment activities. Other documents that may be of assistance are included in the "Further Resources" section of this chapter.)

Communication

Adequate and inclusive communication is an essential component of the emergency response process. Communication should occur between individuals within the organization as well as with those external to the organization. In situations involving an infectious patient(s), direct communication with the local health department must always be included in the initial response. An organization should avoid bypassing its local health department in an effort to speed communications. One of the many responsibilities of the local public health system is to ensure that knowledge is shared with those individuals and organizations that can be of assistance. Failing to adhere to this chain of communication can result in added confusion and interruption of important organizational and agency links. Maintaining a 24-hour contact number for the local health department must be included in emergency response plans.

When addressing the concept of communication, organizations must also consider methods or equipment used in the process. As an organization evaluates existing communication capabilities and develops future plans, representatives from departments that control information systems should be involved. Organizations should recognize that in times of crisis, usual methods of communication may fail, so some consideration of backup measures should be considered and tested.

TIP: *An organizations should avoid bypassing its local health department in an effort to speed communications. One of the many responsibilities of the local public health system is to ensure that knowledge is shared with those individuals and organizations that can be of assistance. Failing to adhere to this chain of communication can result in added confusion and interruption of important organizational and agency links.*

Figure 5-2. Patient Management and Placement for Airborne Precautions: Algorithm

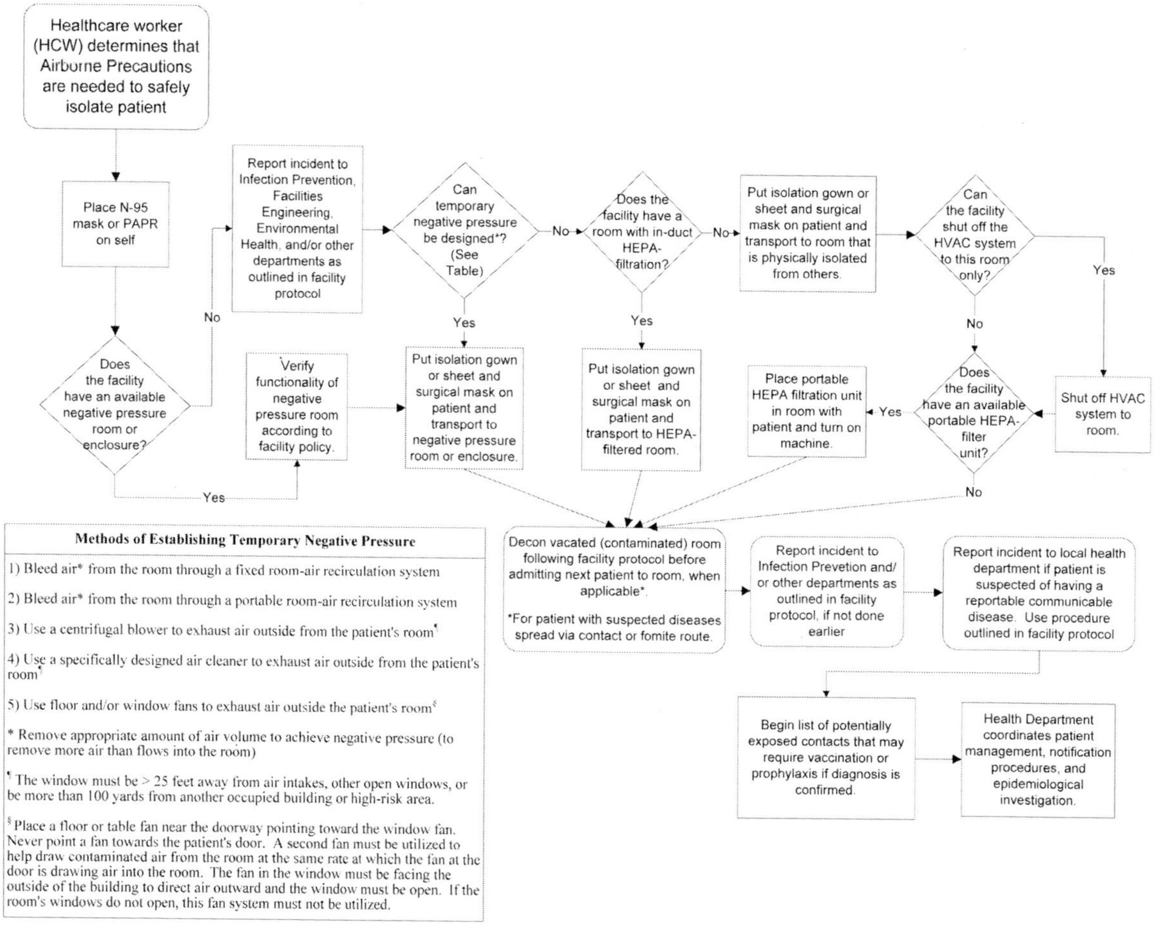

This algorithm shows one approach to managing and placing patients who require airborne precautions. PAPR, powered air purifying respirator; HEPA, high-efficiency particulate air; HVAC, heating, ventilating, and air conditioning.

Source: Adapted from Rebmann T.: Management of patients infected with airborne-spread diseases: An algorithm for infection control professionals. *Am J Infect Control* 33:571–579, Dec. 2005.

Ensuring That Staff Members Are Ready

An emergency situation is not the time to determine whether health care workers are competent to prevent transmission of infection to others or themselves. As previously mentioned, these safe care practices must be part of the daily practice of every health care worker in every health care discipline. Competencies can be defined as a combination of knowledge, attitude, and skills demonstrated by the health care worker.

A set of infection prevention competencies for hospital-based health care workers proposed by Carrico et al. shown in Sidebar 5-2 on page 56. These competencies address the constructs recognition, response, containment, and communication as integral parts of routine, as well as emergency response, practice.

Use of standardization in practices among health care worker disciplines as well as across health care facilities in a given community can assist an infection preventionist in implementing competency-based education. (*See* Sidebar 5-3 on page 56 for education topics—for staff, patients, and visitors—related to emergency management. In addition, an example of isolation signs that have been incorporated into a standardized approach to isolation precautions can be found in Figure 5-3 on page 57.)

Sidebar 5-1: Preparing for an Influx of Infectious Patients Requiring Airborne Infection Isolation

Recognize that an influx of patients requiring an airborne infection illness (negative airflow) environment might exceed current physical plant capabilities. In an effort to begin a planning process, the following information may provide the beginnings of an evaluation process you could include in your emergency preparedness plan. The information noted below is not comprehensive but should serve as a beginning for dialogue with the facility emergency manager, facilities engineering personnel, safety officer, and executive staff:

- Identify existing airborne infection isolation (negative airflow) environments and determine capacity.
- Ensure status of negative airflow using smoke stick or other similar method.
- Evaluate the existing seal of each room. Check seals around windows and electrical outlets.
- Select an appropriate area for surge capacity (wing or separate building), taking the following into consideration:
  — The existing heating, ventilating, and air conditioning (HVAC) system
  — Location of adjacent populations in all directions, especially high-risk areas such as oncology and nurseries
  — Controlled access for traffic patterns
  — Accessibility from areas of first patient encounter (e.g., emergency department, admissions)
  — The existing utility and service capabilities:
    ○ Electrical outlets on emergency backup power
    ○ Oxygen delivery
    ○ Medical gas
    ○ Suction
    ○ Sinks
    ○ Commodes
- Develop a floor plan that indicates blocks of rooms/areas served by each air handler.
- Develop a plan that indicates blocks of rooms/areas served by each ventilation exhaust fan.
- Develop a schematic for each air handling unit (AHU) system indicating flow to each room, return airflow, associated exhaust system, and any recirculation pattern. This information may make you reconsider your initial selection of an appropriate area.
- Identify where air is exhausted and ensure that it is at least 25 feet away from any air intake and 100 yards from other entrances into the facility.
- Evaluate existing equipment, including ventilators, portable suction, and additional oxygen tanks.
- Evaluate existing supplies, including personal protective equipment and suction supplies.

Refer to the algorithm Patient Management and Placement for Airborne Precautions (Figure 5-2) for additional information when attempting to identify additional airborne isolation surge capacity.

Source: Ruth M. Carrico, Ph.D., R.N., C.I.C., Center for Health Hazards Preparedness, University of Louisville School of Public Health and Information Sciences, 2009.

ENSURING THAT THE PHYSICAL PLANT IS READY

Another important consideration for Standard IC.01.06.01 involves the evaluation and capabilities of the physical plant or the care environment and the need to involve the facility's emergency management system early in the process. As was stated earlier, all health care facilities will not need to, or be able to, address this standard in the same manner. Instead, each facility should evaluate its capabilities and role in the community with respect to health care delivery and services.

A thorough evaluation of the limitations and capabilities of the building(s), utilities, ventilation systems, equipment, and supplies will enable planners to determine pockets of need, prioritize activities, and budget for those activities.

Understanding the ventilation system within the physical plant is an important responsibility for an infection preventionist. Figure 5-4, page 65, illustrates a typical patient room and its air distribution system. The figure shows the typical location of supply and return air ducts and the relationship between airflow and patient bed location. Figure 5-5, page 65, shows that a single patient care area is often supplied with air from more than one air handling unit. When investigating appropriate patient placement, ask under what conditions airspace is shared between patients.

Sidebar 5-2: Infection Prevention Competency Statements for Hospital-Based Health Care Workers

1. Describe the role of microorganisms in disease.
2. Describe how microorganisms are transmitted in health care settings.
3. Demonstrate standard and transmission-based precautions for all patient contact in health care settings.
4. Describe occupational health practices that protect the health care worker from acquiring infection.
5. Describe occupational health practices that prevent the health care worker from transmitting infection to a patient.
6. Demonstrate ability to problem-solve and apply knowledge to recognize, contain, and prevent infection transmission.
7. Describe the importance of health care preparedness for natural or manmade infectious disease disasters.

Source: Carrico R., et al.: Infection prevention and control competencies for hospital-based health care personnel. *Am J Infect Control* 36:691–701, Dec. 2008. Used with permission.

Sidebar 5-3: Infection Prevention Education Topics Related to Emergency Management—for Staff, Patients, and Visitors

- Screening/triage procedures (including self-screening for staff during a biological event)
- Patient decontamination procedures
- Patient management (placement/isolation, patient cohorting, transport and discharge protocols, etc.)
- Disease-specific information on bioterrorism agents, emerging infections, and pandemic influenza
- Transmission-based precautions and isolation procedures
- Respiratory etiquette
- Personal protective equipment use and reuse
- Hand hygiene
- Quarantine
- Procedures for obtaining, handling, and processing patient specimens for laboratory testing, including how to coordinate testing through the Laboratory Response Network
- Cleaning and disinfection of toys that are shared between children in the facility
- Procedures during times when visitation is restricted
- Occupational health/safety procedures
- Surge capacity issues that affect infection transmission (e.g., negative pressure surge capacity, lack of personal protective equipment.)
- Organization emergency management plan protocols and procedures that affect infection transmission
- Postmortem care
- Food and water safety, including times when utilities may be not available
- Sanitation control
- Waste management, including times when routine pickup is not available
- Pet management
- Infection prevention protocols for alternative care sites owned/operated by the hospital/health care organization

Source: Adapted from Rebmann T.: APIC state-of-the-art report: The role of the infection preventionist in emergency management. *Am J Infect Control* 37:271–281, 2009. Used with permission.

Figure 5-3. Signage for Isolation Precautions

STANDARD PRECAUTIONS

(If you have questions, go to Nurse Station)

EVERYONE MUST:

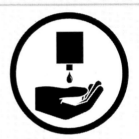 Clean hands when entering and leaving room

Cover mouth and nose with arm or tissue when coughing or sneezing

DOCTORS AND STAFF MUST:

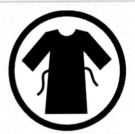 Wear gown and gloves if soiling likely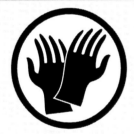

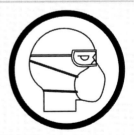 Wear mask and eye cover if splashing body fluids likely

(continued)

Figure 5-3. Signage for Isolation Precautions (continued)

Standard Precautions Routine care that is provided to ALL patients

Family and other visitors to follow precautions.

Hand Hygiene

● Before and after every patient contact, wash or sanitize hands.
● Remove gloves and clean hands when moving from dirty to clean procedures.

Gloves, Gowns, Mask and Eye Protection

Use before coming into contact with non-intact skin, blood, body fluids or secretions.

Personal Protective Equipment:

Put ON in this order:	Take OFF & dispose in this order:
1. **Wash or sanitize hands**	1. Gloves (if used)
2. Gown (if needed)	2. Eye cover (if used)
3. Mask (if needed)	3. Gown (if used)
4. Eye cover (if needed)	4. Mask (if used)
5. Gloves (if needed)	5. **Wash or sanitize hands** (even if gloves used)

Equipment/Supplies:

● Clean and disinfect reusable equipment including IV pumps, cell phone or pagers (if used in room), other electronics, supplies and equipment prior to removing from patient's room.
● Only essential supplies in room.

Room Cleaning:

Routine cleaning procedures with the addition of cubicle curtain changes if visibly soiled.

For any questions contact your hospital's Infection Preventionist.

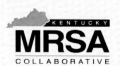

These signs are used to standardize isolation precautions in Kentucky hospitals as part of an MRSA elimination collaborative.

Source: Kentucky MRSA Collaborative. Used with permission.

(continued)

Figure 5-3. Signage for Isolation Precautions (continued)

CONTACT PRECAUTIONS

(If you have questions, go to Nurse Station)

EVERYONE MUST:

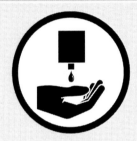

- Clean hands when entering and leaving room

- Follow Standard Precautions

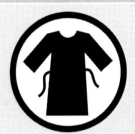 Gown and gloves when entering room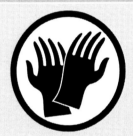

DOCTORS AND STAFF MUST:

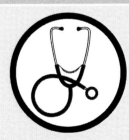

- Use patient dedicated or disposable equipment.

- Clean and disinfect shared equipment.

(continued)

Figure 5-3. Signage for Isolation Precautions (continued)

Contact Precautions

Display sign outside the door. Remove sign _after_ room is cleaned.

Family and other visitors to follow precautions.

Common Conditions:
- Multidrug resistant organisms
  - Methicillin-resistant Staphylococcus aureus (MRSA)
  - Vancomycin-resistant Enterococcus (VRE)
- Clostridium difficile infection (diarrhea)
- Scabies
- Wounds or abscesses with uncontained drainage

Dishes/Utensils:
No special precautions. Kitchenware sanitized in dishwasher.

Equipment and Supplies:
- Use dedicated or disposable equipment when available.
- Clean and disinfect reusable equipment including IV pumps, cell phone or pagers (if used in room), other electronics, supplies and equipment prior to removing from patient's room.
- Ensure blood pressure cuff and stethoscope are cleaned and disinfected between patients.
- Only essential supplies in room.

Linen Management:
Bag linen in the patient's room.

Personal Protective Equipment:

Put ON in this order:	Take OFF & dispose in this order:
1. Wash or sanitize hands	1. Gloves
2. Gown	2. Eye cover (if used)
3. Mask (if needed)	3. Gown
4. Eye cover (if needed)	4. Mask (if used)
5. Gloves	5. Wash or sanitize hands (even if gloves used)

Private Room:
If not available, room with patient that has the same organism but no other infection.

Room Cleaning:
Routine cleaning procedures with the addition of cubicle curtain changes if visibly soiled.

Transport:
Essential transport only. Place patient in clean gown. Clean and disinfect transport vehicle. Alert receiving department regarding patient's isolation precaution status.

Discontinue precautions as per hospital policy or Infection Preventionist instructions.

KENTUCKY
MRSA
COLLABORATIVE

These signs are used to standardize isolation precautions in Kentucky hospitals as part of an MRSA elimination collaborative.

Source: Kentucky MRSA Collaborative. Used with permission.

(continued)

Figure 5-3. Signage for Isolation Precautions (continued)

DROPLET PRECAUTIONS

EVERYONE MUST

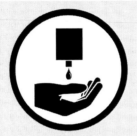
- Clean hands when entering and leaving room

- Follow Standard Precautions

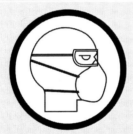
- Wear mask

- Wear eye protection if splash/ spray to eyes likely

DOCTORS AND STAFF MUST

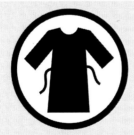
If contact with body fluids likely, use gown, glove, mask and eye protection
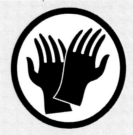

(continued)

Figure 5-3. Signage for Isolation Precautions (continued)

Droplet Precautions

Display sign outside the door. Remove sign after room is cleaned.

Family and other visitors to follow precautions.

Common Conditions:
- Seasonal Influenza
- Bacterial Meningitis (N. meningitidis)
- Pertussis (whooping cough)
- Mumps

Dishes/Utensils:
No special precautions. Kitchenware sanitized in dishwasher.

Equipment and Supplies:
- Use dedicated or disposable equipment when available.
- Clean and disinfect reusable equipment including intravenous pumps, cell phone or pagers (if used in room), other electronics, supplies and other equipment prior to removing from patient's room.
- Ensure blood pressure cuff and stethoscope are cleaned and disinfected between patients.
- Only essential supplies in room.

Linen Management:
Bag linen in the patient's room.

Personal Protective Equipment:

Put ON in this order:
1. Wash or sanitize hands
2. Gown (if needed)
3. Mask
4. Eye cover
5. Gloves (if needed)

Take OFF & dispose in this order:
1. Gloves (if used)
2. Eye cover
3. Gown (if used)
4. Mask
5. Wash or sanitize hands (even if gloves used)

Private Room:
If not available, room with patient that has the same organism but no other infection.

Room Cleaning:
Routine cleaning procedures with the addition of cubicle curtain changes if visibly soiled.

Transport:
Essential transport only and place surgical mask on patient. Clean and disinfect transport vehicle. Alert receiving department regarding patient's isolation precaution status.

Discontinue precautions as per hospital policy or Infection Preventionist instructions.

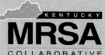

KENTUCKY
MRSA
COLLABORATIVE

These signs are used to standardize isolation precautions in Kentucky hospitals as part of an MRSA elimination collaborative.

Source: Kentucky MRSA Collaborative. Used with permission.

(continued)

Figure 5-3. Signage for Isolation Precautions (continued)

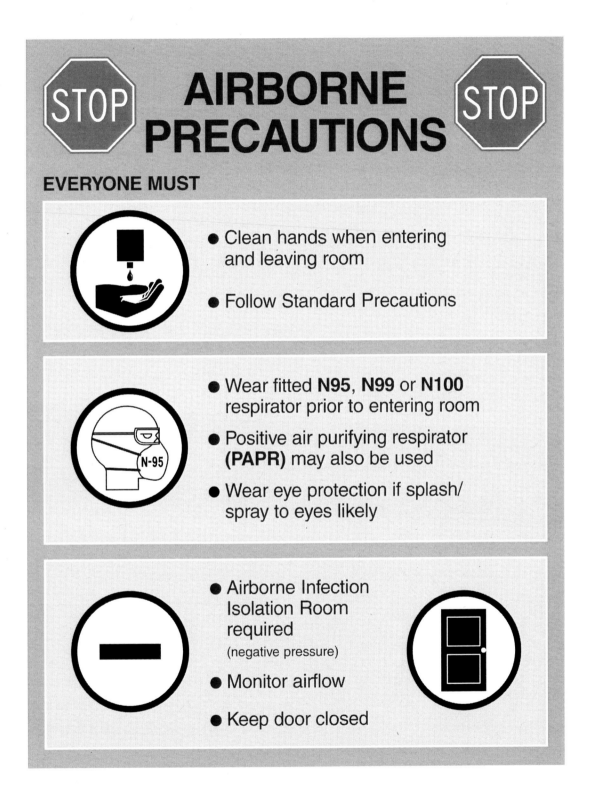

(continued)

Figure 5-3. Signage for Isolation Precautions (continued)

Airborne Precautions

Display sign outside the door. Remove sign after room is cleaned.

Common Conditions:
- Pulmonary or Laryngeal Tuberculosis
- Chicken Pox
- Disseminated Herpes Zoster (shingles)
- Tuberculosis
- Rubeola (measles)
- Avian Influenza

Family and other visitors to follow precautions.

Airborne Infection Isolation Room:
Use airborne isolation room. Nurse to notify Infection Preventionist and Facilities/Engineering of room number when starting and stopping precautions.

Dishes/Utensils:
No special precautions. Kitchenware sanitized in dishwasher.

Equipment/Supplies:
- Use dedicated or disposable equipment when available.
- Clean and disinfect reusable equipment including IV pumps, cell phone or pagers (if used in room), other electronics, supplies and equipment prior to removing from patient's room.
- Ensure blood pressure cuff and stethoscope are cleaned and disinfected between patients.
- Only essential supplies in room.

Linen Management:
Bag linen in the patient's room.

Patient Identification Procedure:
Use patient label for validation of patient identity and destroy in room after use.

Personal Protective Equipment:

Put ON in this order:
1. Wash or sanitize hands
2. Fitted N-95, 99, 100 respirator or PAPR required

Take OFF & dispose outside room, in this order:
1. Fitted N-95, 99, 100 respirator or PAPR required
2. Wash or sanitize hands (even if gloves used)

Room Cleaning:
After patient is discharged, keep door closed for one hour to allow complete room air exchange before routine cleaning procedures. Change cubicle curtain if visibly soiled.

Transport:
Essential transport only and place surgical mask on patient. Clean and disinfect transport vehicle. Alert receiving department regarding patient's isolation precaution status.

Discontinue precautions as per hospital policy or Infection Preventionist instructions.

KENTUCKY
MRSA
COLLABORATIVE

These signs are used to standardize isolation precautions in Kentucky hospitals as part of an MRSA elimination collaborative.

Source: Kentucky MRSA Collaborative. Used with permission.

Figure 5-4. Air Distribution in a Single Patient Room

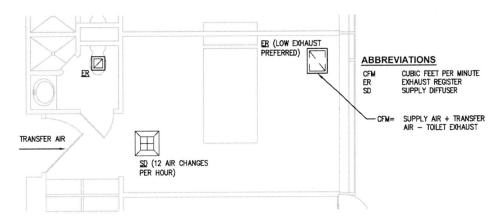

TYPICAL SINGLE OCCUPANCY AIR DISTRIBUTION
(100% OUTSIDE AIR SYSTEM)

This illustration depicts the transfer and exchange of air in a single-occupancy hospital room.

Source: Graphic provided by Jim Hemmer, P.E., Luckett & Farley, Louisville, Kentucky. Used with permission.

Figure 5-5. Schematic of Multiple Air Handlers Servicing a Single Patient Care Area

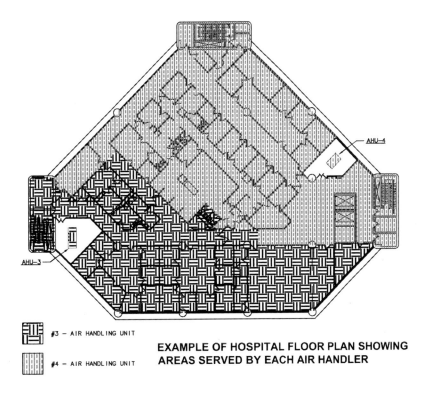

EXAMPLE OF HOSPITAL FLOOR PLAN SHOWING
AREAS SERVED BY EACH AIR HANDLER

This figure depicts the placement of air handling units in a hospital. AHU, air handling unit.

Source: Graphic provided by Jim Hemmer, P.E., Luckett & Farley, Louisville, Kentucky. Used with permission.

EXAMINING OTHER STANDARDS THAT RELATE TO INFECTIOUS DISEASE EMERGENCIES

All Joint Commission standards are designed to form connections with other standards and recognize that there are both complex and complicated linkages and relationships among and between standards. This weaving together of the standards mirrors the comprehensive relationships that must be present and functional as part of the processes of care.

Other standards related to IC.01.06.01 are those that deal with the organization's ability to respond to an emergency. The concepts included in the IC standards support the Joint Commission "Emergency Management" (EM) standards, and both sets of standards serve to continue the focus on the impact infectious patients have on the health care setting and the need to ensure that daily operations support transmission prevention.

Specifically, drills that are part of the EM standards directly link with IC.01.06.01. The existing EM standards require regular drills that test the emergency management responses of the organization. Scenarios that involve infectious agents should be incorporated into an organization's emergency management drill(s) to test the organization's ability to respond to all types of situations. Exercising and evaluating response plans works to protect patients, families, and communities.

APPLYING KNOWLEDGE

Now that the basics of IC.01.06.01 have been reviewed, use the following scenario as a model for how the standard might be met in a given organization and how that organization can demonstrate compliance with the standard's EPs.

The emergency department (ED) charge nurse notifies the nursing supervisor of her concern regarding the number of patients she believes have been seen in the ED during the past several days. To her, it seems that these numbers are growing, and she is noticing that throughput time is increasing. Admissions are slower to be moved from the ED to the nursing care area, and the waiting areas seem to be overburdened with patients exhibiting respiratory symptoms. The nursing supervisor looks at the evening's census and reviews information from the previous several days. She notes that there is a numeric increase in the number of patients seen in the ED with respiratory symptoms but also that there seem to be significantly more patients requiring admission for those symptoms tonight than the night before. Although concerned, she is not alarmed and decides to leave word for the infection prevention department, asking for its immediate input regarding patient placement issues. The tightening of the bed situation has all available private rooms filled, and the charge nurse is also concerned about whether or not each patient has been placed in an appropriate environment. For example, is there a need to house some or all of these patients in an airborne infection isolation (negative airflow) environment?

This case demonstrates a few of the complexities involved in an IPC program. Education of the organizational decision makers (the nursing supervisor), ability to capture information that can be transformed into data that guide decisions (census, syndromic surveillance), early involvement of the infection preventionist(s), and active evaluation of the appropriateness of the care environment and the capabilities of the physical plant are some of the complexities identified in this scenario. Further, this case demonstrates the need to ensure that staff are knowledgeable about and are able to apply infection prevention practice competencies as a routine part of job performance. This involves the ability to think critically and make effective use of limited resources, which may be likely during an actual emergency.

SUMMARY

To comply with IC.01.06.01, organizations must plan for a small-scale (individual organization) and large-scale (communitywide) response. They must engage in comprehensive planning efforts that address the different phases of preparedness, including recognizing, responding to, containing, and communicating about an emergency. Staff must also be familiar with how to control and prevent infections in their daily work and be sensitive to patient issues when they arise. The physical plant must also be ready to respond to an incident involving an influx of infectious patients.

FURTHER RESOURCES

The following sections provide further information on this topic and can serve as a valuable reference in responding to an infectious disease emergency.

CD Tools

The following tools have been provided to offer you examples of thought processes as well as information that can serve as a template for planning efforts. Remember that

Standard IC.01.06.01 does not aim to have all organizations develop similar plans. Instead, the standard aims to have each organization determine its capabilities and its role within its community and to use that information to guide preparedness efforts. The tools address emerging infections as well as agents of bioterrorism.

Tool 5-1: Employee/Occupational Health Considerations

Tool 5-2: Notification Procedures for Health Care Professionals to Report Known or Potential Bioterrorism Incidents: Algorithm

Tool 5-3: Laboratory Testing for Acute, Generalized Vesicular, or Pustular Rash Illness—High Risk: Algorithm

Tool 5-4: Laboratory Testing for Acute, Generalized Vesicular, or Pustular Rash Illness—Low/Moderate Risk: Algorithm

Tool 5-5: Infectious Substance Potential Exposure Response Form

Tool 5-6: Clinical Evaluation of Patients with Possible Inhalational Anthrax: Algorithm

Tool 5-7: Clinical Evaluation of Patients with Possible Cutaneous Anthrax: Algorithm

Tool 5-8: Managing an Exposure to *Bordetella pertussis* (Pertussis, Whooping Cough)

Tool 5-9: Managing an Exposure to Measles Virus (Rubeola)

Tool 5-10: Managing an Exposure to Varicella Virus (Chickenpox)

Tool 5-11: Guide for Preventing Transmission of Selected Infections

Tool 5-12: Guidelines for Reusing Respiratory Protection (N95 Respirators and Surgical/Procedure Masks) During an Infectious Disease Disaster

Web Sites

- American Psychiatric Association (APA): *APA Disaster Psychiatry Materials.* http://www.psych.org/Resources/DisasterPsychiatry/APADisasterPsychiatryResources.aspx.
- Association for Professionals in Infection Control and Epidemiology (APIC) *Bioterrorism Resources.* http://www.apic.org/Content/NavigationMenu/PracticeGuidance/Topics/Bioterrorism/Bioterrorism.htm.
- Canadian Centre for Emergency Preparedness: http://www.ccep.ca.
- Centers for Disease Control and Prevention: *Emergency Preparedness and Response.* http://www.bt.cdc.gov.
- New York State Department of Health: *Emergency Preparedness and Response.* http://www.health.state.ny.us/environmental/emergency/.
- Saint Louis University: *Institute for Biosecurity.* http://bioterrorism.slu.edu.

Additional Readings

- Carrico R. (ed.): *APIC Text of Infection Control and Epidemiology*, 3rd ed. Washington, DC: Association for Professionals in Infection Control and Epidemiology, Inc., 2009.
- Farmer J.C.: *Pandemic Point-of-Care Pocket Guide.* Oakbrook Terrace, IL: Joint Commission Resources: 2007.
- Heymann D. (ed.): *Control of Communicable Diseases Manual*, 19th ed. Washington, DC: American Public Health Association, 2008.
- Homeland Security Council: *Implementation Plan for the National Strategy for Pandemic Influenza.* May 2006. http://www.flu.gov/professional/federal/pandemic-influenza-implementation.pdf.
- Joint Commission Resources: Pandemic preparedness: Best-practice case studies. *Environment of Care News* 10:10–11, May 2007.
- Joint Commission Resources: Preparing for a pandemic: How the Health First hospitals of Brevard County, Florida, developed a pandemic influenza plan. *Environment of Care News* 11:4–10, Jan. 2008.
- *Principles of Disease Transmission.* This Web-based learning opportunity provides free continuing education for nurses. To access, go to http://www.train.org. Log in or create an account and log in. Course ID: 1006060.

- Rebmann T., et al.: *Infection Prevention and Control for Shelters During Disasters*, 2008. http://www.apic.org/Content/NavigationMenu/EmergencyPreparedness/SurgeCapacity/Shelters_Disasters.pdf.
- U.S. Department of Health and Human Services (HHS): *HHS Pandemic Influenza Plan.* 2005. http://www.hhs.gov/pandemicflu/plan/pdf/HHSPandemicInfluenzaPlan.pdf.

- *Virtual Exercise: Unknown Respiratory Illness (for Health Care Professionals).* This virtual exercise is being hosted on the KY TRAIN learning management system. It takes approximately 45 minutes to an hour to complete. To access it, go to http://www.train.org . Login and/or create an account. Course ID: 1014548.

Chapter 6

Interventions and Strategies to Reduce Infection Risk

Loretta L. Fauerbach, M.S., C.I.C.

An infection prevention and control (IPC) plan has to be enacted for change to occur and for the organization's infection prevention program to effectively minimize, reduce, or eliminate the risk of infection.[1,2] Therefore, after performing the risk assessment and developing the IPC plan, the next step in an organization's IPC program is to turn that plan into action. By implementing the right interventions, an organization can improve patient outcomes and reduce infection risks for its patients and employees. Outstanding resources that identify successful interventions and implementation strategies are available through professional associations, health care improvement initiatives, accrediting organizations, and government agencies, as well as the infection control and prevention literature. In addition, many health care organizations have developed a cadre of evidence-based recommendations and implementation strategies and have incorporated these into ongoing practice by monitoring and measuring performance.

An infection preventionist should assemble a comprehensive portfolio of established guidelines and recommendations for the prevention strategies being planned and should consider ways to incorporate improvement strategies into ongoing practice standards. This chapter provides resources for creating strategies for prevention and measuring success. (In addition to those mentioned in the text, refer to the references, resources, and Web sites listed at the end of this chapter.)

STANDARD IC.02.01.01

The [organization] implements its infection prevention and control plan.

STANDARD IC.01.05.01

EP 5

The [organization] describes, in writing, the process for investigating outbreaks of infectious disease.

EXPLORING IC.02.01.01

Standard IC.02.01.01 requires an organization to implement its IPC plan. Although The Joint Commission has identified 10 elements of performance (EPs) for this standard, this chapter addresses only EPs 1, 2, 3, and 5. The other EPs are addressed in Chapters 7 and 8.

IC.02.01.01, EP 1: The [organization] implements the infection prevention and control activities, including surveillance, to minimize, reduce, or eliminate the risk of infection.

The first EP for Standard 02.01.01 is the "umbrella" for all activities related to prevention and control. [*See also* IC.01.05.01, EP 2: *The [organization's] infection prevention and control plan includes a written description of the activities, including surveillance, to minimize, reduce, or eliminate the risk of infection.*] The parameters of this EP are based on the organization's written risk assessment and IPC plan. As discussed in Chapter 4, the risk assessment and IPC plan address the highest infection prevention and control priorities in an organization and those functions that support the IPC program on an ongoing basis. So where does an infection preventionist begin implementation efforts? The following sections aim to answer this question. (*See also* Sidebar 6-1 on page 71.)

Ensure Appropriate Scope for the Infection Prevention and Control Plan

Every organization's IPC program will be different, as it must be based on the unique needs of the organization. That said, an IPC plan must consider specific interventions, including but not limited to the following:

- Improving hand hygiene practices
- Improving cleaning, disinfection, and sterilization practices for equipment, devices, and the environment
- Achieving environmental control through utilities
- Reducing risk associated with maintenance, water, and ventilation
- Implementing standard precautions and transmission-based precautions/isolation
- Preventing surgical site infections
- Preventing device-related infections
- Promoting respiratory etiquette/cough hygiene
- Planning for a bioterrorism event/bioevent and pandemic
- Developing a process to manage outbreaks
- Ensuring occupational health
- Evaluating new and existing products
- Educating staff and patients and their families
- Managing materials (value analysis), including product selection

Based on the assessment of risks and opportunities for improvement, an organization must develop an IPC plan that addresses the areas of key importance to the facility as well as the requirements of the Joint Commission standards, National Patient Safety Goals (NPSGs; *see* Chapter 11) and relevant regulatory and legislative requirements, such as those of the Centers for Medicare & Medicaid Services (CMS). (*See* the "Key Infection Prevention Documents" in the "Further Resources" section of this chapter for more information.)

Implementing Evidence-Based Practices

An infection preventionist's imperative for making sure that patients receive quality care is to ensure that evidence-based guidelines are used to direct that care. Such guidelines should help organizations reach their goal of zero health care–associated infections (HAIs).[2,3]

When considering evidence-based practices, an infection preventionist should refer to the guidelines from the Healthcare Infection Control Practice Advisory Committee (HICPAC) of the Centers for Disease Control and Prevention (CDC) and other CDC documents that provide science-based infection prevention recommendations across the continuum of health care. These recommendations are ranked by category according to the scientific evidence associated with each recommendation, thus providing guidance to the health care provider to assess the minimal and optimal standards that should be met. For example, Category IA, IB, or IC recommendations should be implemented across an organization, because they are based on scientific, epidemiological data or are required by regulations or law.

In addition, many of the HICPAC guidelines include performance measures to assist an infection preventionist in validating a program's compliance. An infection preventionist may want to develop performance measures from the HICPAC documents and other CDC documents (*see* the "Key Infection Prevention Documents" section in the "Further Resources" section of this chapter), including the following:

- *Guideline for Infection Control in Healthcare Personnel*
- *Guideline for Prevention of Surgical Site Infection*
- *Guideline for Environmental Infection Control in Health-Care Facilities*
- *Management of Multi-Drug Resistant Organisms in Healthcare Settings*
- *Guideline for Isolation Precautions: Preventing Transmission of Infectious Agents in Healthcare Settings*
- *Guideline for Disinfection and Sterilization in Healthcare Facilities*

All of these documents are available on the CDC *Infection Control Guidelines* Web page, at http://www.cdc.gov/ncidod/dhqp/guidelines.html.

Professional organizations such as the Association for Professionals in Infection Control and Epidemiology (APIC), the Society for Healthcare Epidemiology of America (SHEA), and the Infectious Diseases Society of America (IDSA) have also championed evidence-based prevention strategies. Multiple publications from these societies are available to assist infection preventionists in guiding and directing the implementation of their organizations' infection prevention programs. For example, APIC's series of elimination guides (http://www.apic.org/eliminationguides) on topics such as *Clostridium difficile,* methicillin-resistant *Staphylococcus aureus* (MRSA), catheter-associated urinary tract infections (CAUTIs), and mediastinitis following cardiac surgery can be helpful. Likewise, the SHEA/IDSA *Compendium of Strategies to Prevent Healthcare-Associated Infections in Acute Care Hospitals*[4] offers many tools and strategies to help with implementation efforts.

In addition to the CDC, APIC, SHEA, and IDSA, the Institute for Healthcare Improvement (IHI) has led major initiatives aimed at reducing HAIs and has obtained the attention of health care providers, administrators, and the public. The IHI is a not-for-profit organization driving the improvement of health care by advancing the quality and value of related practices. Scientific partners with IHI are APIC and SHEA, as well as many other professional organizations. IHI is also working with the CDC and the Joint Commission.

The IHI web site, http://www.ihi.org/IHI, provides comprehensive modules that outline improvement strategies for preventing central line–related infections, ventilator-associated pneumonia (VAP), CAUTI, MRSA, and surgical site infections. There is also a module that addresses hand hygiene improvement.

To formulate its "bundle" approach to prevention, the IHI has incorporated some of the key elements recommended in the HICPAC and APIC guidelines, as well as other infection control literature. It is important to note that only a selected set of recommendations has been included in each bundle. Some Category IA and IB HICPAC recommendations were not included. For example, the IHI VAP bundle is based on having the standard practices recommended by HICPAC already in place for handling tubing, water reservoirs, nebulizers, and other recommendations.[5] It is important for each organization to consider other recommendations and how they may be used when designing prevention strategies based on the IHI bundles. (*See* Tool 6-1, "Tool for Measuring Compliance with IHI Bundles," in the CD Tools section).

Sidebar 6-1. Successfully Implementing Infection Prevention and Control Strategies

Infection prevention and control (IPC) programs that have achieved success in reducing risks for health care–associated infections have used common approaches to implementation, including the following:

1. Team-driven, staff-empowered activities
2. Commitment from administration
3. Involvement of practice leaders as champions
4. Use of consistent and evidenced-based policies and procedures
5. Assurance that needed supplies are readily available to facilitate adherence to recommended practice
6. Requirements for education and competency verification
7. Monitoring and measurement of practices and outcomes via surveillance
8. Effective communication, including feedback of surveillance findings to staff
9. Ongoing evaluation of interventions and continuous improvement activity
10. Interventions hardwired into culture to maintain the gain
11. Celebrations of success.

Developing and implementing strategies to reduce infection risks is a great challenge for IPC programs. Bidirectional communication with all health care providers will help the infection prevention and control team to achieve and sustain effective infection prevention practices. More information on communication can be found in Chapter 7.

TIP: *Health Protection Scotland (HPS) has developed multiple bundles, including a catheter-associated urinary tract infection (CAUTI) prevention bundle with practical examples of checklists and processes to prevent health care–associated infections. The HPS Web site (http://www.hps.scot.nhs.uk/haiic/ic/guidelines.aspx# bundles) provides an example of how to measure compliance with the CAUTI Insertion bundle and how to document the review and assessment of each unit's practice.*

TIP: *Checklists, posters, and reminders are all important tools to facilitate compliance with infection practices. For instance, Saint et al. developed a urinary catheter reminder that was attached to the physician's notes of the chart of each patient who had an indwelling catheter in place for 48 hours.[6] This reminder significantly reduced the catheterization time in the intervention group compared to the control group that did not have a reminder. Incorporating this type of reminder into the management of all devices, not only urinary catheters, can be helpful in decreasing device utilization and associated exposure risks.*

Assigning Responsibility for Implementing Infection Prevention and Control Strategies

As discussed in Chapter 2, it is important to assign responsibility for infection prevention efforts, including responsibility for implementing infection prevention and control strategies. Although designating oversight responsibility is critical, some collaborating groups have recommended that there must also be a personal commitment to implementation from each person involved in prevention initiatives.[7]

Addressing Risks Related to Medical Equipment and Devices

An effective IPC plan must address the provision of safe medical equipment and devices and must ensure appropriate procedures and practices to protect patients and health care staff. Keys to full implementation of the IPC plan are the development and maintenance of comprehensive infection prevention policies and procedures, staff competency in managing devices and equipment, and a mechanism for ensuring that the policies and procedures are consistently followed.

Common themes in all device-related infection prevention activities are identified in Figure 6-1 on page 73. These include the following:

- Supply availability
- Education
- Feedback of outcome and process measures
- Accountability and return demonstration for competency

Interventions to reduce the risks associated with procedures, medical equipment (fixed and portable equipment used for the diagnosis, treatment, monitoring, and direct care of individuals), and medical devices include the following:

- Appropriate storage, cleaning, disinfection, sterilization, and/or disposal of supplies and equipment
- Protocols for reuse of equipment designated by the manufacturer as disposable, in a manner consistent with the manufacturer's instructions and regulatory and professional standards
- Appropriate use of personal protective equipment

Breeches in cleaning and disinfection guidelines, use of unacceptable liquid chemical germicide for disinfection, improper drying, and defective equipment have been responsible for transmission of dangerous pathogens, such as those associated with gastrointestinal endoscopies.[8] The existence of these breeches highlights the need for a health care organization to have a consistent approach to cleaning, disinfection, and sterilization of medical devices. Checklists for determining competency and the use of specific stepwise procedures can facilitate consistency in practice and can be useful as monitoring tools to measure and document compliance. It is important to remember that manufacturer recommendations and material safety data sheets, when applicable, must be included in any checklists of stepwise procedures. (*See* Tool 6-2, "High-Level Disinfection (OPA) Competency Checklist," in the "CD Tools" section.)

Another risk to address regarding medical equipment involves the use of disposable versus reusable equipment. Medical devices are usually labeled by the original manufacturer as either single-use disposable or reusable. It is imperative that the end user understand the difference between these two terms and how to handle a used device based on its designation. An organization must have policies in place to ensure the proper selection, storage, handling, use, and disposition of both reusable and disposable patient care items. If an item can be reprocessed, the manufacturer should provide direction for the approved process. The health care facility should follow those directions and should also set up procedures to monitor the process.

On the other hand, if an item is designated as a single-use disposable item, the item must be discarded after use. The Food and Drug Administration (FDA) has very specific regulations governing the reprocessing of single-use disposable items.[9] If the FDA regulations allow for reuse, the organization may consider establishing an FDA–approved reuse program for the device.

Figure 6-1. 12 Steps in Preventing Device-Associated Infections

1. Use device only when medically necessary according to established criteria.

2. Remove device when it is no longer clinically needed.

3. Implement "bundled care" approach including daily evaluation of whether a patient still needs the device.

4. Use checklist specific for each procedure to ensure compliance with all key bundle components.

5. Monitor practice, assess compliance, and feed back information to all involved in care.

6. Educate health care providers about their role in prevention and use return demonstration to demonstrate competency.

7. Educate patients and families about practices they can use to reduce infection risk.

8. Observe and monitor insertion of all devices and other critical activities.

9. Obtain a commitment from all health care providers to do their part in reducing device-related infections and stress their accountability for adherence to prevention practices.

10. Standardize contents and availability of supplies and kits to facilitate compliance.

11. Perform outcome surveillance for device-associated infection. Report findings to frontline staff, managers, medical staff, and administrators.

12. Promote good hand hygiene and proper sterile and/or aseptic technique.

This figure offers suggested steps to prevent device-associated infections.

Source: Loretta Litz Fauerbach, M.S., C.I.C.

Infection preventionists should be part of the internal evaluation and approval process in determining what devices will be reused. Most hospitals choose to work with an FDA-approved third-party reprocessor. Each third-party reprocessor, including hospitals, must receive FDA approval to reprocess each specific device. It is the responsibility of the organization to confirm that the company it selects meets the FDA regulations for each specific item.[9] (For more information on this topic, *see* Chapter 8.)

Addressing Animals in the Health Care Setting

If an organization uses therapy or service animals in its facility, it must assess and respond to the risks associated with those animals. The therapeutic value of contact with animals is undeniable, and the risks can be minimized with the proper precautions. Animals that enter a health care organization fall into three categories:

1. Service animals
2. Pet therapy animals
3. Personal pets that are brought in to visit their owner

Regardless of the category into which an animal falls, there must be guidelines to ensure patient, personnel, and visitor safety.

Guidelines for animals in the health care setting[10] provide comprehensive information and can provide the basis for health care policies and procedures. For example, the Americans with Disabilities Act of 1990 (ADA) governs service animals that assist their owners. Each health care setting should have a policy that addresses service animals, is consistent with the ADA, and outlines expectations such as grooming, handling, and care provisions for the service animals.

Therapy animals and personal pet visitations are not covered under the ADA but serve important functions in health care settings. Sehulster and Chin address the issues to consider when establishing an animal visitation policy.[11] These include the following:

- Type of animal

- Behavior screening of animal
- Health status
- Management of excreta
- Visitation rules
- The patient's allergies
- Clean up after visitation
- Unit and patient restrictions
- Training of handler

It is particularly important to delineate specific rules and limitations for personal pets that may visit. It may also be prudent to limit personal pets to interactions only with their owners since behavior screening prior to visitation may not be possible. (*See* Table 6-1 on page 75.)

> **TIP:** *It is particularly important to delineate specific rules and limitations for personal pets that may visit. It may also be prudent to limit personal pets to interactions only with their owners since behavior screening prior to visitation may not be possible.*

Considering Surveillance Aspects of the Infection Prevention and Control Plan

As discussed earlier in this publication, surveillance is a key component of an organization's IPC plan. To effectively implement the surveillance aspects of the IPC plan, an organization should have the following items in place:

- A written assessment of the population served, the associated infection risks, and how the organization determined those risks. For example, an analysis of the previous year's data for specific populations or device-related infections, or a list of the high-risk/high-volume procedures and strategies to prevent infections in that arena, would demonstrate compliance. *See* Chapter 4.
- Data that reflect the key outcomes listed in the IPC plan, such as device-related infections or process measures. These data should be reported and available for review. Checklists to illustrate practice compliance can be helpful and can lead to the identification of performance failures.
- The procedure for data collection. The data collection process should also reflect the type of surveillance described in the IPC plan, such as targeted, whole-house, incidence, or prevalence surveillance. Data collection should be accomplished using the definitions

agreed on in the plan. The data should reflect the use of standardized definitions, such as those of the National Healthcare Safety Network (NHSN; http://www.cdc.gov/nhsn/index.html) or those mandated for public reporting.

- Sources of appropriate data needed to identify HAIs
- Descriptions of how to calculate rates
- Methods for analyzing surveillance data

Any reports must be prepared, presented, and distributed to the key stakeholders according to the reporting schedule outlined in the IPC plan. If there is a deviation from the schedule, it is important to note the reasons and what will be done to comply with the schedule in the future.

> **TIP:** *Appropriate laboratory services are key to the success of an IPC program, especially related to surveillance. The laboratory should clearly identify methods used to perform cultures or other tests that identify organisms. The laboratory should identify the limitations of its methodologies so the infection preventionist can evaluate the data and their impact on making clinical decisions. In addition, the laboratory should stay abreast of new technologies related to the identification of emerging pathogens, resistant organisms, and antimicrobial testing.*

IC.02.01.01, EP 2: The [organization] uses standard precautions including the use of personal protective equipment to reduce the risk of infection. (*See also* IC.01.02.01, EP 2.)

IC.02.01.01, EP 2, requires organizations to use standard precautions to reduce the risk of infection and prevent the transmission of pathogens.[12] Such standard precautions include personal protective equipment (PPE) and respiratory and cough etiquette. The following two sections take a closer look at these components.

Personal Protective Equipment

PPE provides barriers for the health care worker to reduce the risk of transmission of bloodborne pathogens, prevent exposure to potentially infectious material, and reduce cross-contamination during patient care activities. The CDC Web site provides posters and guidance on the use of PPE in health care settings (*see* http://www.cdc.gov/ncidod/dhqp/

Table 6-1. Key Considerations for Reducing Risk Associated with Animals in Health Care Settings

KEY CONSIDERATIONS FOR
REDUCING RISK ASSOCIATED WITH ANIMALS IN HEALTH CARE SETTINGS

PEOPLE FACTORS	ANIMAL FACTORS
Education • Handler • Staff • Patient • Family	**Animal Health** • Vaccinations • Flea and tick control • Grooming • Routine care — Feeding — Walking • Zoonotic diseases
Hand Hygiene and Personal Protective Equipment • After animal encounter • Wear gloves to clean up and clean hands after removing gloves when cleaning up animal excreta	**Animal Behavior** • Animal temperament — Predictability of animal type • Transportation • Leash • Crate
Identification of High-Risk Patients • Physician approval • Immunosuppressed patients • Intensive care units and high-risk areas	**Animal Identification** • License • Special garb/kerchief
Environmental Factors Patient room assignment Allergies Hallways Waiting rooms/lounges	**Cleanup and Disposal** • Excreta • Hair shedding, etc.
Policy and Procedures Clear delineation of responsibilities and acceptable practices	

This table shows both animal- and people-related considerations for reducing risks associated with animals in the health care setting.

Source: Loretta Litz Fauerbach, M.S., C.I.C.

index.html). At this site, there are links to the *Workbook for Designing, Implementing, and Evaluating a Sharps Injury Program* and videos, slides, and posters that demonstrate safe use of PPE. Also available at this site, a poster demonstrating the use of PPE is a very helpful aid for teaching how to don and remove PPE. (*See* additional Web site access information at the end of this chapter.)

To reduce the risk of infections, health care organizations should identify the minimal required PPE for protection from risks associated with specific tasks and should provide those supplies. Monitoring PPE use helps ensure staff and patient safety.

This EP also refers to IC.01.02.01, EP 3: *The [organization] provides equipment and supplies to support the infection prevention and control program.* **Note:** *Standard precautions are infection prevention and control measures to protect against possible exposure to infectious agents. These precautions are general and applicable to all patient and residents.* **Footnote:** *For further information regarding standard precautions, refer to the Web site of the Centers for Disease Control and Prevention (CDC) at http://www.cdc.gov.*

Staff members should be able to articulate and demonstrate their competency regarding when and how to use PPE. It is important to understand staff attitudes and knowledge to help design education programs and interventions to improve compliance.[13]

The availability of PPE supplies at the point of use is critical for compliance. Facilities should incorporate an assessment into their process measures for overall compliance with recommended practices this assessment should reflect the availability of supplies as well as the appropriate use of PPE.[12] Each unit or department should be able to demonstrate that it has a mechanism to ensure replacement of supplies when they are low or empty. Noncompliance is often fueled by staff members having to find PPEs when they need them.

TIP: *Staff members should be able to articulate and demonstrate their competency regarding when and how to use PPE. It is important to understand staff attitudes and knowledge to help design education programs and interventions to improve compliance.[13]*

Respiratory Hygiene and Cough Etiquette

Respiratory hygiene and cough etiquette consist of measures to contain respiratory secretions of all individuals who demonstrate signs and symptoms of respiratory infection. These measures are designed to prevent the transmission of respiratory illnesses from people who enter health care settings with cough, congestion, and/or rhinorrhea. To comply with respiratory hygiene and cough etiquette policies, the infected individual must do the following:

1. Cover his or her nose/mouth when coughing or sneezing
2. Use tissues to contain respiratory secretions and dispose of tissues in the nearest waste receptacle after use
3. Clean his or her hands after having contact with respiratory secretions and contaminated objects/materials. This can be accomplished by hand washing with nonantimicrobial or antiseptic soap and water or by using alcohol-based hand rub. (*See the CDC Web site for posters and more information:* http://www.cdc.gov/flu/professionals/infectioncontrol/ resphygiene.htm.)

To help infected individuals use proper respiratory hygiene and cough etiquette, health care facilities must ensure the availability of tissues and hand hygiene supplies. An infection preventionist, in collaboration with other health care providers, should identify where and how to provide access to these critical supplies.

TIP: *Creative signage discussing respiratory hygiene and cough etiquette helps alert visitors and patients to the need for compliance with such hygiene and etiquette. Signs should be placed in the waiting areas and at entrances to the facility to remind everyone about the need to contain respiratory illnesses—such as the flu— and the importance of hand hygiene.*

IC.02.01.01, EP 3: The [organization] implements transmission-based precautions in response to the pathogens that are suspected or identified within the [organization's] service setting and community.

Although standard precautions provide the most basic intervention for preventing transmission of infectious agents during patient care in all health care settings, standard precautions can be enhanced by using transmission-based precautions. These include contact precautions, droplet precautions, and airborne isolation, as recommended in the CDC/HICPAC isolation guidelines for specific infectious agents.[12]

The most current CDC transmission-based isolation guideline is applicable across the continuum of care.[12] Organism-specific infection prevention recommendations are also available from the CDC and others, especially for vancomycin-resistant enterococci (VRE), MRSA,[14] and *Pseudomonas cepacia*.[5] Many states, such as North Carolina and Michigan, also have specific documents regarding the management of multidrug-resistant organisms (MDROs). (*See* "Key Infection Prevention Documents" in the *Further Resources* section in this chapter.)

Each health care setting will have its own unique microbial flora patterns, which reflect its community's and referring institutions' microbiology. Unique concerns often arise in specialized settings such as in intensive care units, long tem care facilities, rehabilitation units, and home health agencies.[15] The emergence of community-acquired MRSA has added another dimension to the complexity of infection prevention and control in all health care settings.[16] An organization should be able to demonstrate how it applies transmission-based practices to prevent transmission of pathogens in its service settings.[17] (More information on this topic can be found in Chapter 11.)

Demonstrating Isolation Strategy Implementation

The successful implementation of isolation strategies can be demonstrated through audits (*see* Tool 6-3, *Compliance Check Sheet for Isolation Precautions*, in the CD Tools) or through surveillance activities that trend the occurrence of epidemiologically significant organisms. For example, increases in acquisition of MDROS may be indicative of noncompliance or system failures with isolation and other infection prevention practices.[18] The ongoing assessment of adherence to appropriate isolation practices, which includes feedback of information to those who can affect practices and the implementation of action plans to improve performance, can be used to demonstrate compliance with IC.02.01.01, EP 3.

An organization might choose to track isolation compliance through graphs reflecting the results of unit-based audits or through demonstration of decreased rates of MDRO acquisition. Improved hand hygiene compliance can also be demonstrated by linking decreasing trends for specific MDROs to improved hand hygiene compliance rates. Graphs demonstrating decreasing trends of central line–associated bloodstream infection (CLABSI) rates can illustrate the success of a performance improvement initiative for preventing CLABSIs. Process measures demonstrating the number of central line insertions that are witnessed and monitored using a checklist versus the total number of central lines inserted can help the infection preventionist determine compliance with this process measure.

IC.02.01.01, EP 5: The [organization] investigates outbreaks of infectious disease. (*See also* IC.01.05.01, EP 5: The [organization] describes, in writing, the process for investigating outbreaks of infectious disease.)

Emerging pathogens have generated much concern among health care providers, public health departments, and the general public for many years.[19] For instance, long noted as an antibiotic-addressed disease, *Clostridium difficile* gained new respect when a more virulent strain emerged and spread in communities, between health care institutions, and worldwide.[20]

At some time in his or her professional career, every infection preventionist will likely have the opportunity and challenge to investigate and control an infectious disease cluster or an outbreak. As discussed in Chapter 5, the scope of the infection preventionist's role in outbreak management involves collaboration with multiple departments in an organization and partnering with public health agencies. Standard IC.02.01.01, EP 5 helps the infection preventionist and the organization be ready to respond to clusters and/or outbreaks. The IPC program must have written documentation outlining how the organization will investigate outbreaks.

Writing the Outbreak Management Plan

An organization can demonstrate compliance with IC.02.01.01, EP 3 by having a written plan that outlines the steps to be taken during an outbreak and that delineates the team members who will be part of the response and their responsibilities. Writing a plan for outbreak management may seem redundant and unnecessary to the infection preventionist, but having a preapproved process will be invaluable during the confusion that often occurs during an outbreak. The written plan will serve as an established road map for the management of the outbreak and ill assist in recruiting needed resources and facilitating administrative approval for the process. Preplanning and education of administrators, managers, and health care workers about the crucial steps in outbreak management will be advantageous in pulling together a team and delineating the processes to be followed in an outbreak situation.

> **TIP:** *The written plan will serve as a preapproved road map for the management of the outbreak and will assist in recruiting needed resources and facilitating administrative approval for the process.*

Primary references for an infection preventionist to use in developing and implementing an outbreak management plan include the two CDC Web site courses listed in the "Further Resources" section of this chapter, the Excite Web site from the CDC (http://www.cdc.gov/excite/classroom/outbreak/index.htm), and Chapter 4, "Outbreak Investigation," from the *APIC Text of Infection Control and Epidemiology.*[21] (*See* further Web site listings for outbreak references and educational materials in "Key Infection Prevention Documents" in the "Further Resources" section of this chapter.)

In addition to developing a written outbreak management plan, an infection preventionist or infection prevention and control department should review the management and identification of any cluster or outbreak after an event and include it in the annual assessment and report. Such a report should describe the event, how it was addressed—including references to the IPC plan—and the actions taken to resolve the problem. The IPC plan should be modified based on any lessons learned from these investigations. In addition, any insights into practice changes or the need for policy changes should be incorporated into the infection prevention and control policies and procedures.

SUMMARY

A critical aspect of any successful IPC program is implementation. Organizations must ensure that the interventions they implement are based on their IPC plans, address risks in the environment, comply with law and regulation, and follow evidence-based practice. This chapter provides many resources for infection preventionists to consult when designing implementation efforts, including efforts related to medical equipment, animal safety, surveillance procedures, standard and transmission-based precautions, and outbreak management.

FURTHER RESOURCES

The following sections provide further information on this topic and can serve as valuable references in implementing a comprehensive IPC program.

CD Tools

Tool 6-1: Tool for Measuring Compliance with IHI Bundles

Tool 6-2: Competency Checklist for Use of High-Level Disinfectant (OPA)

Tool 6-3: Compliance Check Sheet for Isolation Precautions

Key Infection Prevention Documents
APIC Resources

- APIC's Elimination Guides. http://www.apic.org/eliminationguides. This site will host all future elimination guides, as well as those listed here:
  — *Guide to the Elimination of Catheter-Associated Urinary Tract Infections (CAUTIs)*: http://www.apic.org/Content/NavigationMenu/PracticeGuidance/APICEliminationGuides/CAUTI_Guide1.htm
  — *Guide to the Elimination of* Clostridium difficile *in Healthcare Settings.* http://www.apic.org/Content/NavigationMenu/PracticeGuidance/APICEliminationGuides/C_diff_guide.htm.
  — *Guide to the Elimination of Mediastinitis Surgical Site Infections Following Cardiac Surgery.* http://www.apic.org/Content/NavigationMenu/PracticeGuidance/APICEliminationGuides/Mediastinitis_Elimin.htm.
  — *Guide to the Elimination of Methicillin-Resistant* Staphylococcus aureus *(MRSA) Transmission in Hospital Settings.* http://www.apic.org/Content/NavigationMenu/PracticeGuidance/APICEliminationGuides/MRSA_in_Hospital_Set.htm.
  — *Guide to the Elimination of MRSA in Hospital Settings—California Supplement.* http://www.apic.org/Content/NavigationMenu/PracticeGuidance/APICEliminationGuides/MRSA_Guide_CA.htm.
- APIC: *Mandatory Vaccination of Healthcare Workers.* http://www.apic.org/Content/NavigationMenu/GovernmentAdvocacy/IssuesInitiatives/Influenza/HealthcareWorkerImmunization/healthcareimmunize.htm.

- APIC Public Policy and Emergency Preparedness Committees: *APIC Position Paper: Reuse of Respiratory Protection in Prevention and Control of Epidemic- and Pandemic-prone Acute Respiratory Diseases (ARD) in Healthcare,* 2008. http://www.apic.org/Content/ NavigationMenu/EmergencyPreparedness/ PositionPapers/Po.htm .

- Bartley J.M.: The 1997, 1998, and 1999 APIC Guidelines Committees. APIC State-of-the-Art Report: The role of infection control during construction in health care facilities. *Am J Infect Control* 28:156–169, 2000. Available at http://www.apic.org/AM/ Template.cfm?Section=Practice&Template=/CM/HTM LDisplay.cfm&ContentID=11431&MicrositeID=0& WebsiteKey=28980e36-1554-46a7-8e91- d7f06abd0a11.

- Friedman C., et al.: APIC/CHICA–Canada infection prevention, control, and epidemiology: Professional and practice standards. *Am J Infect Control* 36:385–389, 2008. Available at http://www.apic.org/Content/NavigationMenu/ PracticeGuidance/APICCHICAStandards/APIC_ CHICA_Standards.pdf.

- Greene L.R., et al.: *APIC Position Paper: Influenza Immunization of Healthcare Personnel,* Oct. 2008. http://www.apic.org/AM/Template.cfm?Section=Search &section=Position_Statements1&template=/CM/ ContentDisplay.cfm&ContentFileID=11049.

- Sandra L., et al.: Guidelines for animal-assisted interventions in health care facilities. *Am J Infect Control* 36:78–85, 2008. Available at http://www.apic.org/AM/Template.cfm?Template=/CM/ ContentDisplay.cfm&ContentID=12574.

SHEA/IDSA Resources

- Poster on controlling a *C. difficile* outbreak. http://www.rmei.com/cdadposter/ WipeOutCDAD-Poster.pdf.

- SHEA: *Outbreak Resources.* http://www. shea-online.org/news/outbreak_resources.cfm.

- Smith P.W., et al.: SHEA/APIC Guideline: Infection prevention and control in the long-term care facility. *Infect Control and Hosp Epidemiology* 29:785–814, Sep. 2008.

- Yokoe D.S., et al.: A compendium of strategies to prevent healthcare-associated infections in acute care hospitals. *Infect Control Hosp Epidemiol* 29:S1–S92, 2008.

— Editorial. Available at http://www.journals. uchicago.edu/doi/pdf/10.1086/591865.

— Introduction. Available at http://www.journals. uchicago.edu/doi/pdf/10.1086/591063.

— Executive Summary. Available at http://www.journals.uchicago.edu/doi/pdf/10.1086 /591060.

— SHEA/IDSA Practice Recommendation, CLABSIs. Available at http://www.journals. uchicago.edu/doi/pdf/10.1086/591059.

— SHEA/IDSA Practice Recommendation, VAP. Available at http://www.journals.uchicago. edu/doi/pdf/10.1086/591062.

— SHEA/IDSA Practice Recommendation, CAUTIs. Available at http://www.journals.uchicago. edu/doi/pdf/10.1086/591066.

— SHEA/IDSA Practice Recommendation, Surgical Site Infection. Available at http://www.journals. uchicago.edu/doi/pdf/10.1086/591064.

— SHEA/IDSA Practice Recommendation, MRSA. Available at http://www.journals.uchicago. edu/doi/pdf/10.1086/591061.

— SHEA/IDSA Practice Recommendation, *C. difficile.* Available at http://www.journals. uchicago.edu/doi/pdf/10.1086/591065.

The Joint Commission

- *Home page.* http://www.jointcommission.org.

- *Measuring Hand Hygiene Adherence: Overcoming the Challenges.* http://www.jointcommission.org/ NR/rdonlyres/68B9CB2F-789F-49DB-9E3F- 2FB387666BCC/0/hh_monograph.pdf.

- *National Patient Safety Goals.* http://www.jointcommission.org/PatientSafety/ NationalPatientSafetyGoals.

- *National Patient Safety Goals: Easy-to-Read Version.* http://www.jointcommission.org/GeneralPublic/ NPSG/09_npsgs.htm.

IHI Resources

- *How-to Guide: Improving Hand Hygiene.* http://www.ihi.org/IHI/Topics/CriticalCare/ IntensiveCare/Tools/HowtoGuideImproving HandHygiene.htm.

- *How-to Guide: Pediatric Supplement: Reduce Methicillin-Resistant* Staphylococcus Aureus *(MRSA) Infection.* http://www.nichq.org/pdf/FINALMRSA.pdf.

- IHI Central Line bundle. http://www.ihi.org/ IHI/Topics/CriticalCare/IntensiveCare/Changes/ ImplementtheCentralLineBundle.htm.
- IHI UTI bundle. http://www.ihi.org/IHI/Programs/ AudioAndWebPrograms/ExpeditionReducingCatheter AssociatedUrinaryTractInfections.htm.
- IHI Ventilator bundle. http://www.ihi.org/IHI/ Topics/CriticalCare/IntensiveCare/Changes/ ImplementtheVentilatorBundle.htm.

CDC and HICPAC Resources

- Centers for Disease Control and Prevention: Guideline for hand hygiene in health-care settings: Recommendations of the Healthcare Infection Control Practices Advisory Committee and the HICPAC/SHEA/APIC/IDSA Hand Hygiene Task Force. *MMWR Morb Mortal Wkly Rep* 51 (No. RR-16), 2002. Available at http://www.cdc.gov/ncidod/ dhqp/gl_handhygiene.html.
- Centers for Disease Control and Prevention: Guidelines for preventing the transmission of *Mycobacterium tuberculosis* in health-care settings, 2005. *MMWR Recomm Rep* 54:1–141, Dec. 30, 2005. Available at http://www.cdc.gov/mmwr/preview/ mmwrhtml/rr5417a1.htm?s_cid=rr5417a1_e.
- Centers for Disease Control and Prevention, HICPAC: *Guidelines for Preventing Health-Care-Associated Pneumonia, 2003.* Available at http://www.cdc.gov/ ncidod/dhqp/pdf/guidelines/CDCpneumo_guidelines. pdf.
- Centers for Disease Control and Prevention/HICPAC: Guidelines for prevention of intravascular catheter-related infections. *MMWR Recomm Rep* 51(RR10), Aug. 9, 2002. Available at http://www.cdc.gov/ mmwr/PDF/rr/rr5110.pdf. Erratum in *MMWR Morb Mortal Wkly Rep* 51(32), Aug. 16, 2002. Available at http://www.cdc.gov/mmwr/preview/mmwrhtml/mm51 32a9.htm.
- Centers for Disease Control and Prevention: HICPAC. Guidelines for infection control in health care personnel, 1998. *Am J Infect Control* 26: 289–354, 1998. Available at http://www.cdc.gov/ncidod/ dhqp/gl_hcpersonnel.html.
- Centers for Disease Control and Prevention: *Infection Control in Long-Term Care Facilities.* http://www.cdc.gov/ ncidod/dhqp/gl_longterm_care.html.
- Centers for Disease Control and Prevention: *Personal Protective Equipment (PPE) in Healthcare Settings* (videos and slide sets on PPE). http://www.cdc.gov/ncidod/dhqp/ppe.html.
- Centers for Disease Control and Prevention: Poster on PPE. http://www.cdc.gov/ncidod/dhqp/ pdf/ppe/ppeposter1322.pdf.
- Centers for Disease Control and Prevention: Prevention and control of influenza: Recommendations of the Advisory Committee on Immunization Practices (ACIP), 2008. *MMWR Recomm Rep* 57(RR-7):1–60, 2008. Available at http://www.cdc.gov/mmwr/ pdf/rr/rr5707.pdf. Note: The ACIP updates this document annually.
- Centers for Disease Control and Prevention: *Tuberculosis (TB) in Healthcare Settings.* http://www.cdc.gov/ncidod/dhqp/id_tb.html.
- Centers for Disease Control and Prevention: *Workbook for Designing, Implementing, and Evaluating a Sharps Injury Prevention Program*: http://www.cdc.gov/sharpssafety/.
- Division of Healthcare Quality Promotion (DHQP): *Infection Control in Healthcare Settings.* http://www.cdc.gov/ncidod/dhqp/index.html.
- Mangram A., et al.: Guideline for prevention of surgical site infection, 1999. *Am J Infect Control* 27: 97–132, 1999. Available at http://www.cdc.gov/ ncidod/dhqp/gl_surgicalsite.html.
- Rutala W.A., Weber D.J., and the Healthcare Infection Control Practices Advisory Committee: *Guideline for Disinfection and Sterilization in Healthcare Facilities, 2008.* http://www.cdc.gov/ncidod/dhqp/pdf/ guidelines/Disinfection_Nov_2008.pdf.
- Sehulster L., et al.: *Guidelines for Environmental Infection Control in Health-Care Facilities.* 2003. http://cdc.gov/ncidod/dhqp/pdf/guidelines/ Enviro_guide_03.pdf.
- Siegel J.D., et al.: *2007 Guideline for Isolation Precautions: Preventing Transmission of Infectious Agents in Healthcare Settings.* http://www.cdc.gov/ncidod/ dhqp/pdf/isolation2007.pdf.
- Siegel J.D., et al.: *Management of Multidrug-Resistant Organisms in Healthcare Settings, 2006.* http://www.cdc.gov/ncidod/dhqp/pdf/ar/ MDROGuideline2006.pdf.

World Health Organization (WHO)

- *Clean Care Is Safer Care.* http://www.who.int/gpsc/en/.
- Five Moments for Hand Hygiene Poster. http://www.who.int/gpsc/tools/Five_moments/en/index.html.
- *Safe Surgery Saves Lives* (video on safe operating room practices). http://www.who.int/patientsafety/safesurgery/en/index.html.
- *Surgical Safety Checklist.* http://www.who.int/patientsafety/safesurgery/tools_resources/SSSL_Checklist_finalJun08.pdf.
- *WHO Guidelines on Hand Hygiene in Health Care. First Global Patient Safety Challenge: Clean Care Is Safer Care.* http://whqlibdoc.who.int/publications/2009/9789241597906_eng.pdf.

Other Government Sites

- Centers for Medicare & Medicaid Services: *Home page.* http://www.cms.hhs.gov/home/medicare.asp.
- Food and Drug Administration: *Guidance for Industry and FDA Staff—Medical Device User Fee and Modernization Act of 2002, Validation Data in Premarket Notification Submissions (510(k)s) for Reprocessed Single-Use Medical Devices,* 2006. http://www.fda.gov/MedicalDevices/DeviceRegulationand Guidance/GuidanceDocuments/ucm071434.htm.
- National Institute for Occupational Safety and Health (NIOSH): *Recommendations for the Selection and Use of Respirators and Protective Clothing for Protection Against Biological Agents.* NIOSH Publication NO.2009-132, Apr. 2009. http://www.cdc.gov/niosh/docs/2009-132/.
- U.S. Department of Veterans Affairs, Office of Public Health and Environmental Hazards: *Infection: Don't Pass It On.* http://www.publichealth.va.gov/infectiondontpassiton/.

Other Society and Initiative Resources

- American College of Surgeons: *Pay for Performance: Developing a Quality Improvement Framework for Surgical Care.* Sep. 9, 2005. http://www.facs.org/ahp/views/payforperformance.html.
- Brennan K.C., Spitx G.: SCIP compliance and the role of concurrent documentation. *Patient Safety and Quality Healthcare,* Jan./Feb. 2008. http://www.psqh.com/janfeb08/scip.html.

- Health Protection Scotland: http://www.hps.scot.nhs.uk/haiic/ic/guidelines.aspx#bundles.
- Infection Prevention and Control in Pediatric Ambulatory Settings Committee on Infectious Diseases: Policy statement infection prevention and control in ambulatory settings committee on infectious diseases. *Pediatrics* 120:650–665, Sep. 2007. Available at http://pediatrics.aappublications.org/cgi/content/full/pediatrics;120/3/650.
- Nelson D.B., et al.: Multi-society guideline for reprocessing flexible gastrointestinal endoscopes. *Infect Control Hosp Epidemiol* 24:532–537, Jul. 2003. Available at http://www.apic.org/AM/Template.cfm?Section=Guidelines_and_Standards&template=/CM/ContentDisplay.cfm&section=Topics1&ContentID=6381.

Regional and State Organization Resources

- Bartley J., Michigan Society for Infection Control: *Guidelines for Prevention and Control of Antimicrobial Resistant Organisms (ARO). Focus on: Methicillin-Resistant* Staphylococcus aureus *(MRSA) and Vancomycin Resistant Enterococcus (VRE).* 2002. http://www.msic-online.org/resource_sections/aro_guidelines.html.
- Gruden N.: *PRHI Executive Summary.* Pittsburgh Regional Healthcare Initiative, Oct. 2004. http://www.prhi.org/docs/October_2004.pdf.
- Hoffmann K.K., Kittrell I.P.: *Guideline for Control of Antibiotic Resistant Organisms, Specifically Methicillin-Resistant* Staphylococci aureus *(MRSA) and Vancomycin-Resistant Enterococci (VRE).* North Carolina Statewide Program for Infection Control and Epidemiology 1997. http://www.unc.edu/depts/spice/guide.html.
- New Jersey Hospital Association (NJHA), Institute for Quality and Patient Safety: *Antimicrobial Resistance Initiative (AMRI).* http://www.njha.com/qualityinstitute/amri.aspx.
- The Pittsburgh Regional Health Initiative: http://www.prhi.org.

Resources for Outbreak Management

- American Society for Microbiology: MicrobeWorld. http://www.microbeworld.org.

- California Department of Health Services, Division of Communicable Disease Control: Resources and Publications. http://www.cdph.ca.gov/programs/idb/Pages/default.aspx

- Centers for Disease Control and Prevention: *Epidemiology in the Classroom: How to Investigate an Outbreak.* http://www.cdc.gov/excite/classroom/outbreak/objectives.htm.

- Centers for Disease Control and Prevention: *Epi Info.* http://www.cdc.gov/epiinfo/.

- Centers for Disease Control and Prevention: Investigating an outbreak. Lesson 6 in *Principles of Epidemiology in Public Health Practice: An Introduction to Applied Epidemiology and Biostatistics,* 3rd ed. http://www.cdc.gov/training/products/ss1000/ss1000-ol.pdf.

- Colorado Department of Public Health and Environment: *Protocols for Prevention, Treatment and Management of Infectious Diseases for Colorado Long Term Care and Rehabilitation Facilities.* http://www.cdphe.state.co.us/hf/protocols.htm.

- Maryland Department of Health and Mental Hygiene, Office of Epidemiology and Disease Control Programs: *Guidelines: Long Term Care Facilities.* http://www.edcp.org/html/cd_guide.html.

- Ontario Ministry of Health and Long-Term Care, Public Health Division and Long-Term Care Homes Branch: *A Guide to the Control of Respiratory Infection Outbreaks in Long-Term Care Homes.* Oct. 2004. http://www.health.gov.on.ca/english/providers/pub/pub_menus/pub_pubhealth.html.

- Pearce N.: *A Short Introduction to Epidemiology.* Massey University Wellington Campus. http://publichealth.massey.ac.nz/publications/introepi.pdf.

- UCLA Department of Epidemiology, School of Public Health: *John Snow Site.* http://www.ph.ucla.edu/epi/snow.html.

- University of Pittsburgh: *Supercourse: Epidemiology, the Internet and Global Health.* http://www.pitt.edu/~super1/.

- U.S. Food and Drug Administration: *Bad Bug Book.* http://vm.cfsan.fda.gov/~MOW/intro.html.

- WHO: *Weekly Epidemiological Record (WER).* http://www.who.int/wer/en/. This is a good source of global outbreak information.

REFERENCES

1. Pittsburgh Regional Healthcare Initiative puts new spin on improving healthcare quality. *Qual Lett Healthc Lead* 14:2–11, 2002.

2. Gruden N.: *PRHI Executive Summary Report.* Pittsburgh Regional Healthcare Initiative, October 2004. http://www.prhi.org/docs/October_2004.pdf (accessed Oct. 8, 2009).

3. Warye K., Granato J.: Target: Zero hospital-acquired infections. *Healthc Financ Manage* 63:86–91, 2009.

4. Yokoe D.S., et al.: A compendium of strategies to prevent healthcare-associated infections in acute care hospitals. *Infect Control Hosp Epidemiol* 29:S1–S92, 2008.

5. Tablan O.C., et al.: Guidelines for preventing health-care-associated pneumonia, 2003: Recommendations of CDC and the Healthcare Infection Control Practices Advisory Committee. *MMWR Recomm Rep* 53(RR03):1–178, 2004.

6. Saint S., et al.: A reminder reduces urinary catheterization in hospitalized patients. *Joint Commission Journal on Quality and Patient Safety* 31:455–462, 2005.

7. Health Protection Scotland: *Infection Control Health Care Associated Infection Prevention Bundles.* Health Protection Scotland, 2009. http://www.hps.scot.nhs.uk/haiic/ic/guidelines.aspx#bundles (accessed Oct. 8, 2009).

8. Nelson D.B., et al.: Multi-society guideline for reprocessing flexible gastrointestinal endoscopes. *Infect Control Hosp Epidemiol* 24:532–537, 2003.

9. Food and Drug Administration: *Guidance for Industry and FDA Staff—Medical Device User Fee and Modernization Act of 2002, Validation Data in Premarket Notification Submissions (510(k)s) for Reprocessed Single-Use Medical Devices.* Sep. 2006. http://www.fda.gov/MedicalDevices/DeviceRegulationand Guidance/GuidanceDocuments/ucm071434.htm (accessed Oct. 8, 2009).

10. The Writing Panel of the Working Group, et al.: Guidelines for animal-assisted interventions in health care facilities. *Am J Infect Control* 36:78–85, 2008.

11. Sehulster L., Chin R., and Healthcare Infection Control Practice Advisory Committee: Guidelines for environmental infection control in health-care facilities. *MMWR Recomm Rep* 52:1–42, 2003.

12. Siegel J.D., et al.: Guideline for isolation precautions: Preventing transmission of infectious agents in healthcare settings. *Am J Infect Control* 35:S65–S164, 2007.

13. Ellison A.M., Kotelchuck M., Bauchner H.: Standard precautions in the pediatric emergency department: Knowledge, attitudes, and behaviors of pediatric and emergency medicine residents. *Pediatr Emerg Care* 23:877–880, 2007.

14. Bertin M.L., et al.: Outbreak of methicillin-resistant *Staphylococcus aureus* colonization and infection in a neonatal intensive care unit epidemiologically linked to a healthcare worker with chronic otitis. *Infect Control Hosp Epidemiol* 27:581–585, 2006.

15. McGoldrick M., Rhinehart E.: Managing multidrug-resistant organisms in home care and hospice: Surveillance, prevention, and control. *Home Healthc Nurse* 25:580–588, 2007.

16. Jenkins T.C., et al.: Epidemiology of healthcare-associated bloodstream infection caused by USA300 strains of methicillin-resistant *Staphylococcus aureus* in 3 affiliated hospitals. *Infect Control Hosp Epidemiol* 30:233–241, 2009.

17. Gravel D., et al.: Canadian Nosocomial Infection Surveillance Program. Infection control practices related to *Clostridium difficile* infection in acute care hospitals in Canada. *Am J Infect Control* 37:9–14, 2009.

18. Bearman G.M., et al.: A controlled trial of universal gloving versus contact precautions for preventing the transmission of multidrug-resistant organisms. *Am J Infect Control* 35:650–655, 2007.

19. Reingold A.L.: Outbreak investigations: A perspective. *Emerg Infect Dis* 4:21–27, 1998.

20. Baierlein S.A., Wistop A.: *Clostridium difficile. N Engl J Med* 360:636–637, 2009.

21. Checko P.J.: Outbreak Investigation. In Carrico R. (ed.): *APIC Text of Infection Control and Epidemiology*, 3rd ed. Washington, DC: Association for Professionals in Infection Control and Epidemiology, 2009.

Chapter 7

Internal and External Communication Strategies and Mandatory Reporting Requirements

Shannon Oriola, R.N., C.I.C., C.O.H.N.; and Susan M. Slavish, B.S.N., M.P.H., C.I.C.

Effective communication influences all phases of infection prevention and control (IPC) practice. The ongoing, and sometimes urgent, need to communicate information about infections to care providers, related health care organizations, the government, and regulatory agencies requires a thoughtful communication plan that is frequently reviewed, updated, implemented, and monitored.

Lack of communication about infections can create a major barrier to best practices and can ultimately result in negative outcomes for patients and organizations. Conversely, successful communication is not only helpful to those caring for patients but adds value to an infection prevention program, helps reduce the risk of infections and severe infection-related events for patients and staff, and enhances information exchange with leadership and the community.

This chapter discusses how organizations can communicate about infections, focusing on both internal and external reporting requirements. Such requirements may include internal reports to organization leaders, committee members, and staff and external reports to organizations, such as the local or state health department, the National Healthcare Safety Network (NHSN), The Joint Commission, collaborating organizations, and consumers of health care.

TIP: *The ongoing and sometimes urgent need to communicate information about infections to care providers, related health care organizations, the government, and regulatory agencies requires a thoughtful communication plan that is frequently reviewed, updated, implemented, and monitored.*

REPORTING AND COMMUNICATING ABOUT INFECTIONS

Effective communication can weave threads of continuity and clarity throughout a health care organization and can yield a number of positive dynamics, including collaboration, cooperation, and teamwork. The Joint Commission requires organizations—through the Joint Commission "Leadership" standards—to create and maintain a culture of safety based on open communication. (*See* Chapter 3.) Key components of a culture of safety are transparency of information and effective communication about such information.

As organizations move toward cultures based on transparency and open communication, the need for effective reporting of and communication about infections is paramount. Both internal and external communication are necessary in a comprehensive IPC program. Open communication is a powerful tool in preventing health care–associated infections (HAIs) and fostering a safe environment.

There are many ways organizations can communicate about infections that may assist in fostering a culture of patient safety and minimize or eliminate infections. These different ways include, but are not limited to, the following:

- Informing direct patient care providers about the number and identity of patient(s) who acquired particular infections, such as *Clostridium difficile*-infections, on their units each month
- Providing information to modify physician behavior for improved compliance with an organization's infection prevention protocols
- Empowering patients to speak up when health care providers fail to wash their hands or clean an injection

- port prior to intravenous (IV) medication administration
- More information on these methods of communication, as well as others, follows

---

STANDARD IC.02.01.01

The [organization] implements its infection prevention and control plan.

EXPLORING IC.02.01.01

Within Joint Commission Standard IC.02.01.01, there are five elements of performance (EPs 7 through 11) related to communication and reporting requirements. The following sections take a close look at these EPs and provide suggestions for compliance.

IC.02.01.01, EP 7: The [organization] implements its methods to communicate responsibilities for preventing and controlling infection to licensed independent practitioners (LIPs), staff, visitors, patients, and families.

The time of entry into an organization provides an excellent opportunity to communicate an individual's responsibility for preventing and controlling infection (whether that individual is a patient, staff member, licensed independent practitioner, or volunteer). Examples of entry points where information can be shared include new employee and volunteer orientation, the process a physician goes through to obtain privileges or when beginning a new internship or residency, and patient or resident admission to the facility.

Educating Staff

Most, if not all, organizations include information on preventing infection during new staff orientation. This information can be delivered via face-to-face presentations, self-learning modules, videos, written materials, or computer-based education. These same methods are also effective for conveying information when introducing an educational topic to existing employees, such as how to prevent central line–associated bloodstream infections (CLABSIs).

Writing an article for the physician newsletter or attending meetings with physician groups to provide an update on infection prevention issues is often an effective communication strategy for reaching physicians. In-services or courses offering continuing medical education (CME) credit pro-

vided by the health care organization or an affiliated university have also been successful in educating physicians about infection prevention.

METHODS FOR EDUCATING STAFF ABOUT INFECTIONS
- Face-to-face presentations
- Self-learning modules
- Videos
- Written materials
- Computer-based education
- Newsletter articles
- Continuing medical education courses

Educating Patients

To educate patients about infection, many health care facilities have created a patient or resident safety brochure or use the patient safety brochure on preventing infections available from the Joint Commission (see http://www.jointcommission.org/PatientSafety/SpeakUp). This brochure describes five things patients and families can do to prevent infection, including washing their hands and making sure health care providers wash their hands. A patient safety brochure about preventing infection is typically given to a patient upon admission to the hospital or other health care setting.

In addition to a patient safety brochure, special patient education materials can be developed for a variety of infection prevention issues, such as preventing the spread of influenza, ensuring proper wound care, and safely using urinary catheters. These materials can be produced in various languages and can include graphics. They can also be designed to address the learning needs of different patient populations.

The Joint Commission is not the only organization that provides patient education materials about infections. Other organizations, including the Society for Healthcare Epidemiology of America (SHEA), the Association for Professionals in Infection Control and Epidemiology (APIC), the Centers for Disease Control and Prevention (CDC), and the Institute for Healthcare Improvement (IHI), have developed pamphlets and brochures to assist in educating patients and their families on the prevention of HAIs. (*See* Figure 7-1 on page 87.) Organizations may want to consider using these materials in their patient education efforts.

Figure 7-1. Example of a Patient Guide on Health Care–Associated Infection

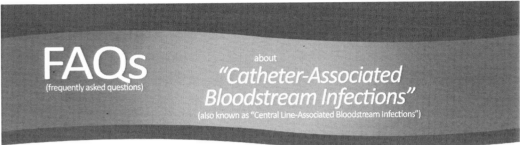

FAQs (frequently asked questions) about "Catheter-Associated Bloodstream Infections" (also known as "Central Line-Associated Bloodstream Infections")

What is a catheter-associated bloodstream infection?

A "central line" or "central catheter" is a tube that is placed into a patient's large vein, usually in the neck, chest, arm, or groin. The catheter is often used to draw blood, or give fluids or medications. It may be left in place for several weeks. A bloodstream infection can occur when bacteria or other germs travel down a "central line" and enter the blood. If you develop a catheter-associated bloodstream infection you may become ill with fevers and chills or the skin around the catheter may become sore and red.

Can a catheter-related bloodstream infection be treated?

A catheter-associated bloodstream infection is serious, but often can be successfully treated with antibiotics. The catheter might need to be removed if you develop an infection.

What are some of the things that hospitals are doing to prevent catheter-associated bloodstream infections?

To prevent catheter-associated bloodstream infections doctors and nurses will:
- Choose a vein where the catheter can be safely inserted and where the risk for infection is small.
- Clean their hands with soap and water or an alcohol-based hand rub before putting in the catheter.
- Wear a mask, cap, sterile gown, and sterile gloves when putting in the catheter to keep it sterile. The patient will be covered with a sterile sheet.
- Clean the patient's skin with an antiseptic cleanser before putting in the catheter.
- Clean their hands, wear gloves, and clean the catheter opening with an antiseptic solution before using the catheter to draw blood or give medications. Healthcare providers also clean their hands and wear gloves when changing the bandage that covers the area where the catheter enters the skin.
- Decide every day if the patient still needs to have the catheter. The catheter will be removed as soon as it is no longer needed.
- Carefully handle medications and fluids that are given through the catheter.

What can I do to help prevent a catheter-associated bloodstream infection?

- Ask your doctors and nurses to explain why you need the catheter and how long you will have it.

- Ask your doctors and nurses if they will be using all of the prevention methods discussed above.
- Make sure that all doctors and nurses caring for you clean their hands with soap and water or an alcohol-based hand rub before and after caring for you.

If you do not see your providers clean their hands, please ask them to do so.

- If the bandage comes off or becomes wet or dirty, tell your nurse or doctor immediately.
- Inform your nurse or doctor if the area around your catheter is sore or red.
- Do not let family and friends who visit touch the catheter or the tubing.
- Make sure family and friends clean their hands with soap and water or an alcohol-based hand rub before and after visiting you.

What do I need to do when I go home from the hospital?

Some patients are sent home from the hospital with a catheter in order to continue their treatment. If you go home with a catheter, your doctors and nurses will explain everything you need to know about taking care of your catheter.

- Make sure you understand how to care for the catheter before leaving the hospital. For example, ask for instructions on showering or bathing with the catheter and how to change the catheter dressing.
- Make sure you know who to contact if you have questions or problems after you get home.
- Make sure you wash your hands with soap and water or an alcohol-based hand rub before handling your catheter.
- Watch for the signs and symptoms of catheter-associated bloodstream infection, such as soreness or redness at the catheter site or fever, and call your healthcare provider immediately if any occur.

If you have additional questions, please ask your doctor or nurse.

Co-sponsored by:

One way to educate patients and families on how to prevent health care–associated infections is to use the six *Patient Guides on Healthcare-Associated Infections* developed by the Society for Healthcare Epidemiology of America's (SHEA's) Patient Safety and Quality Improvement Committee in collaboration with the Centers for Disease Control and Prevention. These brochures can be given to patients when discussing prevention of the infections addressed in SHEA's *Compendium of Strategies to Prevent Healthcare-Associated Infections in Acute Care Hospitals.* The Compendium and Patient Guides are available online at http://www.shea-online.org/about/compendium.cfm. This figure shows one of the six guides.

Source: Society for Healthcare Epidemiology of America (SHEA), Arlington, Virginia. Used with permission.

IC.02.01.01, EP 8: The [organization] reports infection surveillance, prevention, and control information to the appropriate staff within the [organization].

There are a variety of ways to communicate information about infection surveillance, prevention, and control to the appropriate staff. For example, infection control committee members can communicate with staff. The infection control committee is typically made up of key leaders and staff in the organization who need to know how the program is performing. These members use their expertise and experience to make recommendations for improvement. They are also responsible for sharing relevant data and information with the staff in the departments they represent and with staff and physicians who provide direct patient care, where appropriate.

Communication of information about infection prevention or regarding a practice change may also be sent through a governance structure of several key committees. These might include a patient safety and quality improvement group, senior executives, or the governing board. Reporting may also occur through a clinical practice council composed of direct patient care providers who receive information, make decisions, and are responsible for reporting the results of these decisions back to their units. By sharing information at the council level, decisions made by staff can provide insight into best strategies for success and barriers that may prevent achievement of successful outcomes.

Real-time notification via e-mail to the clinical manager—to be shared with staff—or making rounds on a unit can be helpful. For example, rounds on a unit where a patient develops a CLABSI can be powerful, particularly if staff investigate the possible causes of the infection and share a reminder of best practices with caregivers to prevent further CLABSIs.

Another effective way to communicate with direct patient care providers is to use a unit-specific dashboard of key infection performance indicators, updated monthly, that includes items such as HAIs that occur on that unit and unit-specific hand hygiene compliance. An example of a dashboard is provided in Figure 7-2, page 89.

With successful communication, direct patient care providers begin to rely on data to make decisions regarding thier practice and behaviors, which can ultimately reduce the incidence of HAIs. For example, the National Nosocomical Infections Surveillance (NNIS) system (now the NHSN) has been able to demonstrate reduction in CLABSI rates when data are disseminated to health care providers and there is an association between the reduced rates and successful prevention interventions (*see* Figure 7-3, page 89).[1]

An article published in February 2009 reprinted that a decline in the incidence of methicillin-resistant *Staphylococcus aureus* (MRSA) CLABSIs was observed in most U.S. intensive care units (ICUs) reporting to the CDC from 1997 through 2007.[2] This article demonstrates that continued data feedback to clinicians combined with a focus on infection prevention efforts resulted in a decrease in CLABSIs in organizations reporting data to the CDC.

Furthermore, in an article by Assanasen, Edmond, and Bearman, assessing compliance with infection prevention practices in two ICUs, the authors concluded that the following:

> Feedback of infection control process measures and major HAIs to unit leadership significantly improved compliance with head of bed (HOB) elevation rates and Foley catheter (FC) use but not hand hygiene (HH). Multilevel feedback significantly improved HH compliance and delivered a satisfactory level of compliance with HOB and FC use in both ICUs during the study period.[3]

Because providing data can help change practice, communicating information regarding infection prevention and control to physicians, interns, and residents is essential in academic or integrated health care settings where physicians may be hired by the hospital and in community hospitals where the physicians are on the medical staff roster but are not employed by the organization. Providing feedback directly to physicians regarding specific outcomes, such as their own specific surgical site infection rate(s), has been demonstrated through the Study of the Efficacy of Nosocomial Infection Control (SENIC) Project[4] to be effective in reducing HAIs. For example, sending a letter to both the surgeon and anesthesiologist when the prophylactic antibiotic is not administered within 60 minutes prior to the initial incision can be helpful in improving compliance with recommended surgical prophylaxis practice (*see* example in Figure 7-4 on page 90).

Figure 7-2. Infection Control Dashboard

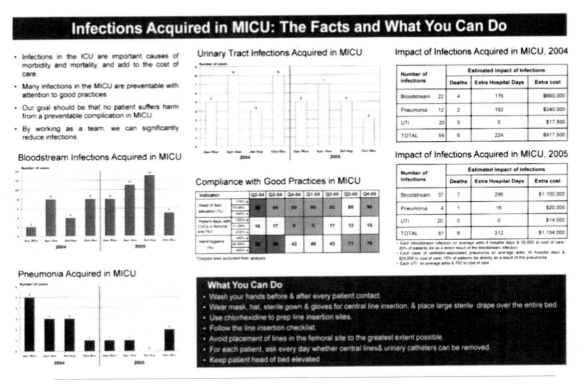

This example of a dashboard from the Virginia Commonwealth University (VCU) Medical Center shows one way the organization communicates with staff about infections.

Source: Virginia Commonwealth University Medical Center, Richmond, Virginia. Used with permission.

Figure 7-3. Trends in Bloodstream Infection Rates by Type of Intensive Care Unit, National Nosocomial Infections Surveillance System, 1990–1999

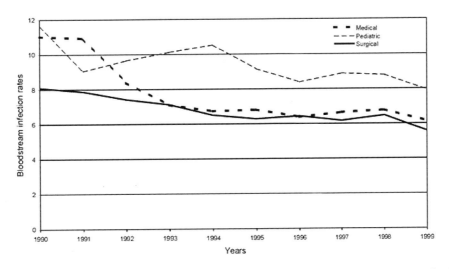

This figure shows a positive correlation between reduced bloodstream infection rates and data dissemination to health care providers.

Source: Gaynes R., et al.: Feeding back surveillance data to prevent hospital-acquired infections. *Emerg Infect Dis* 7:295, 298, Mar.–Apr. 2001. Used with permission.

Figure 7-4. Example of a Letter to a Physician on Timeliness of Preoperative Prophylactic Antibiotic Administration

SHARP MEMORIAL HOSPITAL

INFECTION SURVEILLANCE AND CONTROL PROGRAM

To:	Dr. _____
From:	_____ Hospital Epidemiologist _____ Medical Director, Orthopedic and Spine Service Lines
Subject	*Timeliness of Pre-operative Prophylatic Antibiotic Administration*
Date:	

Correct timing of pre-operative prophylactic antibiotic administration decreases the risk of surgical site infections (see graph below). The IDEAL is to start the administration of cephalosporins and clindamycin within 60 minutes and vancomycin within 120 minutes of incision.

Regulatory agencies now review this data to ascertain optimal patient care.

The Orthopedicand Anesthesiology Supervisory Committees have requested that we provide feedback to orthopedic and spine surgeons and anesthesiologists should their patient not have received their prophylatic agent on time. Unless there is **DOCUMENTATION** of receipt of the prophylatic agent, we will have to assume that the agent was not given. The following information is tabulated for your review.

Patient	MR#	Date of Surgery	Antibiotic	Time infusion started	Time of Incision	Anesthesiologist

**Timing of Prophylatic Antibiotics and
Surgical Site Infection Rates**

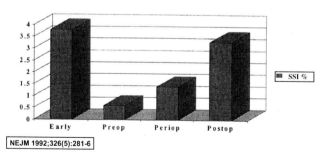

NEJM 1992;326(5):281-6

Thank you for your attention to this matter.

This letter is used to communicate with physicians to help improve compliance and change practice.

Source: Sharp Memorial Hospital, San Diego, California. Used with permission.

IC.02.01.01, EP 9: The [organization] reports infection surveillance, prevention, and control information to local, state, and federal public health authorities in accordance with law and regulations.

IC.02.01.01, EP 9, represents one of the most fundamental epidemiologic practices of infection prevention and control. Reporting information regarding patients with communicable diseases, such as AIDS or tuberculosis, to the local public health department is essential in preventing the spread of the diseases to others in the community and is required by law or regulation in all states.

Outbreaks in health care facilities, such as those caused by a norovirus or scabies, should also be reported to the local health department and/or the state licensing and certification division. The CDC can assist in outbreak investigation, particularly if the severity in patient outcomes is significant and the cause of the outbreak is difficult to determine. The Division of Healthcare Quality Promotion (DHQP) of the CDC will respond to an outbreak investigation only when specifically asked by a state department of public health services.

Although local and state laws have required the reporting of communicable diseases and outbreaks for decades, recent legislation in many states requires the reporting of HAI data to a state agency, often with subsequent reporting to the public. What must be reported is very different from state to state, and only a handful of states have been able to share the information with the public at this time. Most states use the NHSN definitions and methodology to determine whether an infection is associated with care and treatment that was provided by a health care organization. As of mid-2009, more than 20 states required HAIs to be reported to the NHSN (*see* http://www.apic.org for more information), and several other states had pending legislation for reporting.

In addition to reporting HAI rates to the state and the public, some states now require either implementation of a program to reduce HAIs related to MRSA or an active surveillance testing program to detect MRSA colonization. Health care organizations in these states must demonstrate compliance with program requirements and/or must report data on active surveillance test results.

IC.02.01.01, EP 10: When the [organization] becomes aware that it transferred a patient who has an infection requiring monitoring, treatment, and/or isolation, it informs the receiving organization.

In most hospitals in the United States, case managers or discharge planners assist with the placement of patients who will subsequently require medical care or treatment in a variety of health care settings. Once the appropriate facility has been selected and the patient has been accepted, the case manager or discharge planner is responsible for communicating the treatment plan and any relevant information for the patient. This includes information such as an infection that continues to require antibiotic therapy and the precautions the organization took to prevent spread of the infection to others. Figure 7-5 on page 92 is an example of one method that can be used to communicate this information.

IC.02.01.01, EP 10, also requires organizations to measure the success of the process of information reporting to the receiving organization. Auditing the communication form that the discharge planner completes is one way to determine whether the appropriate information was shared prior to discharge of the patient. An organization can also maintain a log (in paper or electronic form) to demonstrate communication of important patient care issues to receiving organizations.

There are times when a culture result indicating infection is reported after the patient has been discharged from the organization. Communicating final laboratory results of a bloodstream infection or wound infection to the attending physician or receiving health care facility may expedite appropriate antibiotic therapy for the patient. If the organism is multidrug resistant, facility policy may require the patient to be placed in contact precautions.

In some organizations, the reporting of infections post discharge to the receiving facility is a responsibility of a number of team members. A log maintained by an infection preventionist (or an other professional) who records the name of the receiving facility and the laboratory result reported, will meet the intent of IC.02.01.01, EP 10. An example of a log is given in Figure 7-6, page 93.

Figure 7-5. Example of Discharge Planner Communication of Infection/Isolation

SHARP. Memorial Hospital

TODAY'S DATE: _____

PATIENT NAME: _____ REFERRED BY: _____
DOB: _____ AGE: _____ PHONE: _____ PAGER: _____
SEX: _____ PRIMARY LANGUAGE: _____ CURRENT PT. LOCATION: _____
HT: ___'___" WT: ___lbs._____ ATTENDING MD: _____
ACUTE ADMIT DATE: _____ PRIMARY MD: _____
ANTICIPATED TRANSFER DATE: _____ MD TO FOLLOW AT SNF: _____
CODE STATUS:☐ FULL CODE ADV. DIR. YES NO INSURANCE: _____
            ☐ DNR
HOSPITAL DISCHARGE DIAGNOSIS: _____
SURGERIES WITH DATES: _____
SIGNIF. MEDICAL HISTORY: _____
_____

PRIOR LIVING SITUATION: _____
ANTICIPATED DISCHARGE TO: _____
FAMILY CONTACT PERSON: _____ PHONE: _____ EXT _____

MENTAL STATUS   MEDICATIONS   BOWEL: _____
___ALERT/ORIENTED   ___PO   BLADDER: _____
___FORGETFUL   ___NG/PEG
___CONFUSED   ___IV   DIET: _____
___COMATOSE   (NAME/DOSE/FREQ)   ___SELF   ___TPN
                          _____   ___ASSIST ___TUBE
BEHAVIOR   _____   TF FORMULA: _____
___COOPERATIVE   _____   TUBE TYPE: _____
___AGITATED
___NOISY   ┌──────────────────────┐
___COMBATIVE   _____   │ RESPIRATORY CARE   │
RESTRAINTS   IV ACCESS TYPE AND LOCATION │ O2_____ TRACH____ │
                         _____   │ TREATMENTS _____ │
SITTER_____   SKIN (LOCATION/TREATMENT) │ SUCTION FREQ._____ │
REASON_____   INCISIONS: _____   └──────────────────────┘

┌──────────────────────┐ _____   ┌──────────────────────┐
│ PSYCHOTROPIC MEDS: │   │ INFECTIONS   │
│ (Med/Dose/Routine/PRN)│ TEARS: _____   │ SITE_____ │
│   │   │ INF AGENT_____ │
│ _____   │ PRESSURE SORES: _____   │ ISOLATION_____ │
│ _____   │ _____   └──────────────────────┘
│ _____   │ _____   ┌──────────────────────┐
└──────────────────────┘ _____   │ DIABETES CARE   │
                         _____   │ ROUTINE INSULIN_____ │
ACTIVITY ASSIST LEVELS_____ _____   │ SLIDING SCALE_____ │
BED MOB: _____ _____   │ FREQ. OF TEST_____ │
TRANSFERS: _____ _____   │ BS RANGE_____ │
GAIT:_____ SPECIAL BED TYPE:_____   │ BEDREST_____ │
__PHYSICAL THERAPY __OCCUPATIONAL THERAPY __SPEECH THERAPY └──────────────┘
THERAPY OF NOTES: _____   ┌──────────────────────┐
_____   │ DIALYSIS (TYPE/SCHED.)│
_____   │ _____   │
                                                  └──────────────────────┘

HX OF FALLS AT HOME OR IN HOSPITAL

_____
_____   ┌──────────────────────┐
___CHEST XRAY:_____   │ ALLERGIES: │
COMMENTS: _____   │   │
_____   └──────────────────────┘
_____
_____

This tool helps ensure the effective exchange of information between organizations.

Source: Sharp Memorial Hospital, San Diego, California. Used with permission.

TIP: *Communicating final laboratory results of a bloodstream infection or wound infection to the attending physician or receiving health care facility may expedite appropriate antibiotic therapy for the patient.*

IC.02.01.01, EP 11: When the [organization] becomes aware that it has received a patient from another organization who has an infection requiring action, and the infection was not communicated by the referring organization, it informs the referring organization. *Note:* Infections requiring action include those that require isolation and/or public health reporting or those that may aid in the referring organization's surveillance.

While investigating a possible HAI during routine surveillance, it sometimes becomes apparent that the infection originated at another health care organization. For example, a

patient may have total hip arthroplasty at one facility but have incision and debridement of the surgical site infection at another facility, or scabies may be diagnosed after a resident has been transferred from a skilled nursing facility to the hospital. In these cases, if the infection was unknown to the referring organization at the time of transfer, the referring organization would benefit from being informed of the diagnosis so it could then investigate other possible cases and interrupt further transmission of infection.

Given the constant flow of patients and residents between facilities and inpatient and outpatient settings, having reciprocal arrangements with external organizations that frequently send or receive patients is important. One approach to ensuring effective communication across settings is for organizations that regularly transfer patients to each other to develop agreements or memorandums of understanding regarding this reporting process to ensure consistency in practice and a flow of information that will benefit the patients and protect health care workers.

Figure 7-6. Communication Log

Referring organization	Infection and associated pathogen (device/procedure)	Patient name and date of birth	Date facility notified	Person notified

This is an example of a log kept for notifying referring health care organizations of a patient who has an infection that requires action.

Source: Shannon Oriola, R.N., C.I.C., C.O.H.N.

SUMMARY

This chapter looks at how organizations can communicate about infections. It discusses the need to be open and transparent with staff, licensed independent practitioners, volunteers, and patients about infections and their roles in preventing infections. In addition, the chapter discusses the need to report infections—those resulting from communicable diseases, HAIs, outbreaks, and so forth—to local, state, and federal authorities as well as to internal sources, such as the infection control committee. When transferring patients from one care setting to another, organizations must also communicate about infections and be sure to document that communication appropriately.

REFERENCES

1. Gaynes R., et al.: Feeding back surveillance data to prevent hospital-acquired infections *Emerg Infect Dis* 7:295, 298, Mar.–Apr. 2001.

2. Burton D., et al.: Methicillin-resistant *Staphylococcus aureus* central line–associated bloodstream infections in US intensive care units, 1997–2007. *JAMA* 301:727–736, 2009.

3. Assanasen S., Edmond M., Bearman G.: Impact of 2 different levels of performance feedback on compliance with infection control process measures in 2 intensive care units. *Am J Infect Control* 36: 407–413, Aug. 2008.

4. Haley R.M., et al.: Efficacy of infection surveillance and control programs in preventing nosocomial infections in US hospitals. *Am J Epidemiol* 121:182–205, Feb. 1985.

Chapter 8

The Environment of Care and Infection Prevention and Control

Kathleen Meehan Arias, M.S., C.I.C.; and Barbara Moore Soule, R.N., M.P.A., C.I.C.

The Joint Commission's "Infection Prevention and Control" (IC) standards and "Environment of Care" (EC) standards both aim to promote a safe, functional, and supportive environment. They also stress the importance of a proactive, systematic approach to managing infection risks. For example, the IC and EC standards require identification and management of infection risks related to the following:

- Building design, construction, and renovation
- Medical equipment, devices, and supplies
- Utility systems
- Infectious waste

Organizations are expected to engage in ongoing efforts to provide a safe environment and to ensure immediate interventions when conditions result in a threat to life or health. This chapter examines the role of the environment of care in infection prevention and control (IPC) efforts and offers suggestions on how to ensure a safe, functional, and supportive environment that effectively manages infection risks.

TIP: *Organizations are expected to engage in ongoing efforts to provide a safe environment and to ensure immediate interventions when conditions result in a threat to life or health.*

THE IMPACT OF THE ENVIRONMENT ON INFECTION PREVENTION AND CONTROL EFFORTS

Because the health care environment—especially contaminated air, water, and medical devices—can serve as a source of pathogenic organisms, the IPC program risk assessment should address the role that the environment contributes to

infection risk in the organization. Based on the risk assessment, the IPC program should identify and implement measures that will reduce the risk of transmission or acquisition of organisms from environmental sources to patients, residents, staff, or visitors and should monitor compliance with those measures.

One aspect of the environment that should receive attention from the IPC program is the role of environmental surfaces in transmitting disease. Although the role of environmental surfaces, furnishings, carpeting, laundry, plants, and medical waste in disease transmission in health care facilities is limited,[1] some human pathogens—such as vancomycin-resistant Enterococci (VRE), norovirus, hepatitis B virus, and *Clostridium difficile*—can remain infective on environmental surfaces for prolonged periods.[1] Therefore, protocols for cleaning and disinfecting environmental surfaces, furnishings, and medical equipment and devices, as well as for handling linens and waste are integral components of the IPC program.[1]

Outbreaks associated with contaminated environmental surfaces have been reported. For example, norovirus outbreaks in the health care setting have been associated with touching contaminated surfaces and a lack of subsequent hand hygiene. One norovirus outbreak at a tertiary care center required closure of patient care units and disinfection of the environment to stop an outbreak that lasted three months, caused illness in 90 patients and 255 health care workers, and cost an estimated $657,644.[2]

In addition to environmental surfaces, the following have also contributed to serious outbreaks in health care settings and are well documented in the literature[1]:

- Construction, renovation, and alteration of the physical facility
- Contamination of the water supply
- Inadequate ventilation

STANDARD IC.02.01.01

The [organization] implements its infection prevention and control plan.

EP 6: The [organization] minimizes the risk of infection when storing and disposing of infectious waste.

STANDARD IC.02.02.01

The [organization] reduces the risk of infection associated with medical equipment, devices, and supplies

STANDARD EC.02.04.03

The [organization] inspects, tests, and maintains medical equipment.

STANDARD EC.02.05.01

The [organization] manages risks associated with its utility systems.

STANDARD EC.02.06.01

The [organization] establishes and maintains a safe, functional environment.

STANDARD EC.02.06.05

The [organization] manages its environment during demolition, renovation, or new construction to reduce risk to those in the organization.

STANDARD EC.04.01.01

The [organization] collects information to monitor conditions in the environment.

STANDARD EC.04.01.05

The [organization] improves its environment of care.

Note: *Not all of these standards apply to all types of health care settings. An organization should consult its current* Comprehensive Accreditation Manual *to determine applicability.*

EXPLORING THE "INFECTION PREVENTION AND CONTROL" AND "ENVIRONMENT OF CARE" STANDARDS

Although many of the EC standards can be applied to infection prevention and control activities, this chapter focuses only on the following IC and EC topics:

- Infectious waste
- Medical equipment, devices, and supplies
- Sterilizers
- Hemodialysis water
- Utility systems
- Environmental services and housekeeping
- Demolition, renovation, and construction
- Monitoring and improving conditions in the environment

The following sections take a closer look at the IC and EC standards that address these topics and provide practical strategies and interventions to help organizations and infection preventionists provide a safe environment, prevent infections, and meet the requirements of the standards and their elements of performance (EPs).

IC.02.01.01, EP 6: The [organization] minimizes the risk of infection when storing and disposing of infectious waste. (*See also* EC.02.02.01, EP 1.)

The intent of IC.02.01.01, EP 6, is to ensure that health care organizations have developed and implemented safe systems and processes to dispose of infectious waste from the time it is generated, such as at the bedside, to the time it leaves the facility, to final disposal.

An infection preventionist can help ensure that IC.02.01.01, EP 6, is met by assessing the organization's practices and policies for collecting, storing, and disposing of infectious waste (also called *regulated medical waste*) and by ensuring that these policies are in compliance with local, state, and federal requirements. Such assessment can occur when the infection preventionist performs the annual infection prevention and control risk assessment and conducts environmental tours.

Most regulations related to infectious or regulated medical waste are defined at the state level, usually by the state health department. These requirements typically address the following topics:

- Treatment
- Storage
- Transportation
- Transfer facilities
- Packaging and labeling of potentially infectious waste

An infection preventionist must identify the applicable requirements and collaborate with staff in the organization who generate and manage infectious waste to ensure compliance with those requirements.

Information on some state requirements can be found on the Environmental Protection Agency (EPA) Web site at http://www.epa.gov/osw/nonhaz/industrial/medical/programs.htm. The Occupational Safety and Health Administration (OSHA) also addresses the issue of infectious waste and specifies certain features of regulated waste containers—including appropriate tagging—to protect personnel against exposure to bloodborne pathogens.[3] However, the ultimate disposal method (landfilling, incinerating, and so forth) for infectious waste falls under the purview of the EPA and state and local agencies.[4]

TIP: *An infection preventionist can maintain current information about infectious waste requirements by joining health department mailing lists, linking to the appropriate Web sites for updated information, and maintaining a close relationship with others in the organization who may receive this information on a regular basis.*

In addition to assessing policies and practices, an infection preventionist should also evaluate health care workers' compliance with accepted practices by performing environmental rounds, documenting findings, and sending a report to the units surveyed.

STANDARD IC.02.02.01

The [organization] reduces the risk of infection associated with medical equipment, devices, and supplies.

Requirements for managing medical equipment, devices, and supplies are included in both the EC and IC standards. This section addresses the IC Standard requirements, and the following section examines the EC requirements. Note that there are several links between many of the EPs of different standards related to medical equipment, devices, and supplies.

IC.02.02.01, EP 1: The [organization] implements infection prevention and control activities when doing the following: cleaning and performing low-level disinfection of medical equipment, devices, and supplies.

Note: *Low-level disinfection is used for items such as stethoscopes and blood glucose meters. Additional cleaning and disinfecting is required for medical equipment, devices, and supplies used by patients/residents who are isolated as part of implementing transmission-based precautions.*

For further information regarding cleaning and performing low-level disinfection of medical equipment, devices, and supplies, refer to the Web site of the Centers for Disease Control and Prevention (CDC), at http://www.cdc.gov/ncidod/dhqp/sterile.html.

The risk of infection from medical equipment and devices that have contact with intact skin, such as stethoscopes, pulse oximetry sensors, and blood pressure cuffs, is low.[1] However, because these items readily become contaminated during use and are potential sources for transmission, organizations should have policies for cleaning and disinfecting them using a low-level disinfection protocol, in accordance with manufacturer instructions, recognized standards, and the organization's procedures.[1]

IC.02.02.01, EP 2: The [organization] implements infection prevention and control activities when doing the following: performing intermediate and high-level disinfection and sterilization of medical equipment, devices, and supplies. (*See also* Standard EC.02.04.03, EP 4.)

Note: *High-level disinfection is used for items such as respiratory equipment and specula. Sterilization is used for items such as implants and surgical instruments. High-level disinfection may also be used if sterilization is not possible, as is the case with flexible endoscopes.*

For further information regarding performing intermediate and high-level disinfection of medical equipment, devices, and supplies, refer to the Web site of the Centers for Disease Control and Prevention (CDC), at http://www.cdc.gov/ncidod/dhqp/ sterile.html.

Medical devices that come into contact with mucous membranes or nonintact skin are known as semicritical items and must receive high-level disinfection, at a minimum.[1] Examples are bronchoscopes, endoscopes, specula and respiratory therapy equipment such as ventilators. Medical instruments or devices that contact normally sterile areas of the body or enter the vascular system are known as critical items.[1] Because there is a high risk of infection from such devices if they are microbiologically contaminated, they must be sterilized before use.[1] These items include surgical instruments, cardiac catheters, implants, and ultrasound probes used in sterile body cavities.

TIP: *The services or departments responsible for cleaning, disinfecting, and sterilizing medical equipment, devices, and supplies should have clear policies and procedures based on knowledge, experience, guidelines from respected organizations, and best practices.*

An organization can provide a safe environment and can demonstrate compliance with this standard by taking the following actions:

- Developing and implementing cleaning, disinfection, and sterilization protocols based on recognized standards and recommendations, such as those from the Association of PeriOperative Registered Nurses (AORN), the Association for the Advancement of Medical Instrumentation (AAMI), and the Centers for Disease Control and Prevention (CDC)[5–7]
- Implementing a mechanism for classifying reusable medical equipment and devices as noncritical, semicritical, or critical and identifying how they will be processed between patients
- Using multidisciplinary teams to develop and implement standardized policies and procedures for handling, cleaning, disinfecting, sterilizing, and disposing of or storing medical equipment, devices, and supplies.
- Ensuring that cleaning, disinfection, and sterilization practices are standardized and implemented consistently throughout the organization.
- Ensuring availability of policies and procedures that are consistent with manufacturer recommendations and recognized practices[5–7] and that include the following:

- *Who* (for example, housekeeper, central service worker, nursing assistant, nurse) is responsible for cleaning and disinfecting/sterilizing items
- *What* cleaning and disinfecting products should be used (for example, quaternary ammonium compound, phenolic, bleach)
- *Where* cleaning and disinfecting/sterilizing efforts should occur (for example, patient room, soiled utility room, central processing)
- *When* cleaning and disinfecting/sterilizing should occur (for example, after each use, prior to removing from a patient room, daily)
- *How* cleaning and disinfecting/sterilizing should occur

- Providing orientation, training, and competency programs for staff involved in cleaning, disinfecting, and sterilizing medical equipment, devices, and supplies
- Developing, implementing, and monitoring quality assurance protocols for high-level disinfection and sterilization processes. For example, such protocols must address the use of chemical indicators, administrative controls, and biological monitors for sterilizers and chemical test strips to evaluate the concentration of high-level disinfectants such as glutaraldehyde or peracetic acid.[5–7]
- Conducting quality assurance monitoring for high-level disinfection and sterilization processes, in accordance with manufacturer recommendations and recognized standards and recommendations, such as those from the AORN, AAMI, and CDC[5–7]
- Creating and implementing a specific recall protocol that can be activated if performance monitoring or other findings indicate that the sterilization process fails[7]
- Ensuring adequate staffing levels and supervision of personnel who process medical equipment, devices, and supplies
- Developing and implementing a system for assessing personnel adherence to cleaning, disinfection, and sterilization protocols and feeding back findings to these personnel
- Ensuring availability of policies and procedures for repair or disposal and, if indicated, replacement of damaged equipment and devices

Another related standard is IC.01.04.01, EP 4: The [organization's] written infection prevention and control goals include the following: limiting the transmission of infections associated with the use of medical equipment, devices, and supplies. *This goal should be considered in the IPC risk assessment. (For more information, see Chapter 4.)*

An infection preventionist should work with other organization staff to ensure that there is consistency among all areas that perform medical equipment and instrument cleaning, disinfection, sterilization, and disposal or storage procedures. In addition, an infection preventionist should receive reports of quality assurance tests that indicate that the sterilization process likely failed and the follow-up that was done.

IC.02.02.01, EP 3: The [organization] implements infection prevention and control activities when doing the following: disposing of medical equipment, devices, and supplies.

An organization can demonstrate compliance with IC.02.02.01, EP 3, when health care workers dispose of medical equipment, devices, and supplies according to established policy. For those items that are contaminated or considered infectious waste, staff members should follow the disposal policy that addresses contaminated or infectious waste disposal and that complies with applicable regulations. Those items that are considered noninfectious or regular waste can usually be discarded in the regular waste stream.

IC.02.02.01, EP 4: The organization implements infection prevention and control activities when doing the following: storing medical equipment, devices, and supplies.

To prevent supplies from becoming contaminated or compromised during storage, infection preventionists should work with staff to ensure that medical equipment, devices, and patient care items are stored appropriately, in protected areas with controlled traffic flow. In addition, infection preventionists should make sure that staff members are knowledgeable about storing these items.

Some further issues to consider regarding storing medical equipment, devices, and supplies include the following:
- Shelving used to store equipment, devices, and supplies, and the areas around and under the shelving, must be cleanable.
- There should be a process in place to determine whether items are clean and intact prior to use and to ensure that packaging has not been torn or punctured.
- Each organization should determine whether it will use a

time-limited or event-related process for rotating supplies.
- Circumstances under which expired items are discarded should be clearly defined, and staff should be clear about these processes.

IC.02.02.01, EP 5: When reprocessing single-use devices, the [organization] implements infection prevention and control activities that are consistent with regulatory requirements and professional standards.

Inappropriate reprocessing of single-use devices (SUDs) can compromise patient safety. The U.S. Food and Drug Administration (FDA) has strict requirements for reprocessing devices labeled for single use under the Federal Food, Drug, and Cosmetic Act.[8] The FDA requires that reprocessors of these devices provide validation data that include cleaning and sterilization data and functional performance data demonstrating that each SUD will remain substantially the same after the maximum number of times the device is reprocessed. (Third-party reprocessors can be used to meet these requirements.) In other words, before a device that is intended for one use or use on a single patient during a single procedure can be reprocessed and reused, a third party or hospital must comply with the same requirements that apply to original equipment manufacturers.

To meet IC.02.02.01, EP 5, the infection preventionist should collaborate with personnel in patient care and reprocessing areas to ensure that SUDs, especially those used in invasive procedures, are not reprocessed and reused unless the organization can meet the FDA requirements.[8] Because most health care organizations cannot meet these rigorous requirements, the majority either use a third-party reprocessor that can meet the requirements or choose not to reprocess and reuse SUDs.

Additional information about reprocessing SUDs can be found on the FDA Web site using the search term "single use device" (http//www.fda.gov) and in the "Further Resources" section of this chapter.

STANDARD EC.02.04.03

The [organization] inspects, tests, and maintains medical equipment.

Like Standard IC.02.02.01, Standard EC.02.04.03 illustrates the importance of medical equipment maintenance and testing in infection prevention and control efforts, specifically the maintenance and testing of sterilizers and hemodialysis equipment.

EC.02.04.03, EP 4: The [organization] conducts performance testing of and maintains all sterilizers. These activities are documented. (*See also* IC.02.02.01, EP 2.)

The machinery used to sterilize devices, equipment, and supplies used for patient care must work effectively so that the organization can ensure that each item processed is safe for patient care. To comply with EC.02.04.03, EP 4, an organization must have documentation that performance testing—including mechanical, chemical, and biological monitoring—is conducted on all sterilizers in accordance with manufacturer recommendations and standardized, accepted practices.[5-7]

In collaboration with the staff members who use sterilizers, infection preventionists should review sterilizer performance monitoring and maintenance records to ensure that maintenance is occurring and that sterilizers are working properly.

EC.02.04.03, EP 5: The [organization] performs equipment maintenance and chemical and biological testing of water used in hemodialysis. These activities are documented.

Because contaminated water and improperly processed equipment can result in adverse patient reactions and death, it is critical that the water and practices used in hemodialysis are safe.[9-11] To prevent adverse events and comply with EC.02.04.03, EP 5, each setting that performs hemodialysis should have the following:

- Clear policies and procedures and strict controls on managing the water supply, which are based on recognized standards and recommendations[1,12]
- A program for regularly conducting chemical and biological testing of water used in the hemodialysis process and documenting the results[1,12]
- A system for reviewing the results of chemical and biological testing, which includes the assignment of responsibility for review and follow-up to a designated person. There should be evidence that abnormal results are immediately investigated and corrective measures are taken, as appropriate.
- For further information on this topic, the AAMI provides standards for dialysis water purity and water distribution and storage systems,[12] and the CDC's

Guidelines for Environmental Infection Control in Health-Care Facilities provides an overview of dialysis water quality and dialysate.[1]

EC.02.05.01: The organization manages risks associated with its utility systems.

In addition to medical equipment, an organization's utilities can present opportunities for pathogenic growth and transmission. The following sections discuss two aspects of utility systems of which infection preventionists should be aware.

EC.02.05.01, EP 5: The [organization] minimizes pathogenic biological agents in cooling towers, domestic hot- and cold-water systems, and other aerosolizing water systems.

Water, aqueous solutions, water systems, and moist environments can serve as sources and reservoirs for pathogenic agents. Environmental reservoirs and sources for microbial pathogens include the following[1]:

- Cooling towers and evaporative condensers
- Dialysis water and equipment
- Ice machines and ice
- Hydrotherapy tanks and pools
- Equipment that is connected to main water systems, such as endoscope reprocessors and dental unit water lines

Because of the potential for pathogens associated with water in the environment, infection preventionists should be familiar with the basic components of water systems in health care facilities, the modes of transmission for waterborne infectious diseases that have been transmitted in health care facilities, and strategies for preventing and controlling waterborne microbial transmission, acquisition, and contamination.[1] Such strategies can include the following:

- Contingency plans for provision of potable water during periods of contamination or disruption
- Implementation of a surveillance program to detect health care–associated infections resulting from *Legionella* species[1,13]
- A program for inhibiting the growth of *Legionella* species in the potable water system and in cooling towers (*see* http://www.Legionella.org)
- A program for maintaining and monitoring dialysis system water and dialysate quality[1,12]
- Adherence to AAMI standards for hemodialysis[12]

- A risk assessment for *Legionella* species in cooling towers and potable water (Risk assessment tools are available from the State Government of Victoria, Australia, Department of Human Services, at http://www.health.vic.gov.au/environment/legionella/industry.htm.)

TIP: *Because of the potential for pathogens associated with water in the environment, infection preventionists should be familiar with the basic components of water systems in health care facilities, the modes of transmission for waterborne infectious diseases that have been transmitted in health care facilities, and strategies for preventing and controlling waterborne microbial transmission, acquisition, and contamination.[1]*

EC.02.05.01, EP 6: In areas designed to control airborne contaminants (such as biological agents, gases, fumes, dust), the ventilation system provides appropriate pressure relationships, air-exchange rates, and filtration efficiencies.

Note: *Areas designed for control of airborne contaminants include spaces such as operating rooms, special procedure rooms, delivery rooms for patients diagnosed with or suspected of having airborne communicable diseases (for example, pulmonary or laryngeal tuberculosis), patients in "protective environment" rooms (for example, those receiving bone marrow transplants), laboratories, pharmacies, and sterile supply rooms. For further information, see Guidelines for Design and Construction of Hospitals and Health Care Facilities, 2001 edition, published by the American Institute of Architects.[13]*

Heating, ventilating, and air conditioning (HVAC) systems can serve as reservoirs and sources of pathogenic organisms and have been involved in disease transmission in health care facilities.[1] Infection preventionists should become familiar with the airborne infectious diseases that have been transmitted in health care facilities and the basic components and operations of HVAC systems. To do this, infection preventionists should consider reviewing publications about HVAC systems and infectious diseases associated with those systems,[1,13–16] attending educational programs, and working with their organizations' facilities and maintenance personnel.

TIP: *The* Guidelines for Design and Construction of Hospitals and Health Care Facilities *address indoor air-quality standards, including ventilation rates, temperatures, humidity levels, pressure relationships, and minimum air changes per hour specific to different areas of health care facilities. This can be a useful resource when learning about HVAC systems and the infection prevention and control issues associated with them.*

Strategies for complying with EC.02.05.01, EP 6, include the following:

- Developing and implementing policies and procedures for ensuring the proper maintenance and functioning of HVAC systems in the facility
- Documenting routine monitoring of the functioning of air-handling systems in special care areas—such as airborne infection isolation areas, protective environments, and operating rooms. Documentation should also include steps that are taken if the system is not functioning according to established criteria.[13,14]
- Ensuring the prevention and control of infection during demolition, construction, and renovation activities (*see* the discussion of Standard EC.02.06.05)

EC.02.06.01: The [organization] establishes and maintains a safe, functional environment.

As previously mentioned, the role of environmental surfaces—such as floors, walls, furnishings, sinks, carpets, and curtains—is limited in disease transmission in health care facilities.[1] Nevertheless, it is imperative that cleaning and disinfecting protocols for these surfaces be in place throughout a health care facility. Such environmental services and housekeeping protocols should effectively reduce the bioburden on environmental surfaces to lessen the likelihood that they could serve as a source for pathogenic agents. Such protocols should also ensure an aesthetically pleasing environment for patients, residents, visitors, health care personnel, and others.

Strategies for addressing environmental services and housekeeping issues include the following:

- Ensuring collaboration between infection prevention and control and environmental services personnel to develop and implement policies and procedures for cleaning and disinfecting environmental surfaces and handling laundry and medical waste (including sharps)[1]

- Conducting a risk assessment to identify and focus on appropriate care of high-touch surfaces—such as bedrails and the area around toilets in patients' or residents' rooms[1]
- Fostering collaboration between infection prevention and control and environmental services personnel to ensure that appropriate cleaning and disinfecting agents are used and that they do not damage the surfaces on which they are used
- Providing ongoing training and monitoring of environmental services personnel to ensure that they use appropriate practices and types and concentrations of cleaners and disinfectants
- Using a multidisciplinary team approach to conducting routine rounds to evaluate environment-of-care issues, such as cleanliness, storage of supplies, eating and drinking on care units, and management of medical devices and equipment. (Tools 8-3, 8-6, 8-9, and 8-10—found in the "CD Tools" of this chapter—provide sample environmental rounds forms.) Members of a multidisciplinary environmental rounds team could include personnel from infection prevention and control, environmental services, nursing services, facilities maintenance, safety, and performance improvement.

TIP: *Environmental services and housekeeping protocols should effectively reduce the bioburden on environmental surfaces to lessen the likelihood that they could serve as a source for pathogenic agents. Such protocols should also ensure an aesthetically pleasing environment for patients, residents, visitors, health care personnel, and others.*

EC.02.06.05: The [organization] manages its environment during demolition, renovation, or new construction to reduce risk to those in the organization.

> **STANDARD EC.02.06.05**
> EP 1: When planning for new, altered, or renovated space, the [organization] uses one of the following design criteria:
> - State rules and regulations
> - *Guidelines for Design and Construction of Hospitals and Health Care Facilities*, 2001 edition, published by the American Institute of Architects

> - When the above rules, regulations, and guidelines do not meet specific design needs, other reputable standards and guidelines that provide equivalent design criteria (*See also* EC.02.05.01, EP 1.)
> EP 2: When planning for demolition, construction, or renovation, the organization conducts a preconstruction risk assessment for air quality requirements, infection control, utility requirements, noise, vibration, and other hazards that affect care, treatment, and services.
> EP 3: The organization takes action based on its assessment to minimize risks during demolition, construction, or renovation.

Strategies for providing a safe environment and complying with requirements for building design, demolition, construction, and renovation include the need to do the following:

- Form a multidisciplinary, collaborative team to identify and proactively mitigate the effects of demolition, construction, and renovation activities on air quality, water and HVAC systems, environmental cleanliness, and traffic flow. This team must include the infection preventionist, and other members may include experts in facility design and ventilation, safety officers, epidemiologists, building engineers, direct care supervisors, risk managers, and building contractors.
- Document when infection preventionists are actively involved in a health care facility's planning, design, demolition, construction, and renovation. Proof of involvement could include sign-off on planning and design documents or infection prevention and control construction permits.
- Identify and use applicable state and local regulations and other relevant requirements when designing, renovating, and constructing new health care facilities.
- Use the *Guidelines for Design and Construction of Hospitals and Health Care Facilities* when designing and planning new spaces and renovating existing ones.[14]
- Complete a preconstruction risk assessment, including an infection control risk assessment (ICRA), which incorporates risk criteria for evaluating the type of activity that will occur and the types of patients who will be affected during construction and renovation projects.[1,13] Issues to assess during a preconstruction risk assessment include the following:
  - Disruption of essential services

- Relocation or placement of patients
- Barrier placements to control airborne contaminants
- Debris cleanup and removal
- Traffic flow

(Tool 8-1, found in the "CD Tools" section of this chapter, provides an example of an ICRA.)

- Use an infection control permit for demolition, construction, and renovation activities. This is a tool that can be used to document and communicate with the contractor about his or her responsibilities regarding the preconstruction risk assessment and to document follow-up visits by the infection preventionist or safety manager. (An example of an infection control permit can be found in Tool 8-2 in the "CD Tools" section of this chapter.)

- Use barriers, high-efficiency particulate air (HEPA) filtration units, and other measures to create negative pressure in the construction space and prevent the dispersion into occupied areas of airborne organisms and dust particles produced by construction and renovation activities.

- Monitor and document daily the presence of negative airflow within the construction zone or renovation area.[1] (An example of a monitoring form can be found in the "CD Tools" section of this chapter.)

- Develop and implement a comprehensive IPC program during maintenance, demolition, construction, and renovation projects.

- Implement a multidisciplinary program for training, monitoring, and promoting adherence to infection prevention and control practices during construction and renovation.

EC.04.01.01: The organization collects information to monitor conditions in the environment.

STANDARD EC.04.01.01

EP 12: The [organization] conducts environmental tours every six months in patient care areas to evaluate the effectiveness of previously implemented activities intended to minimize or eliminate environment of care risks. (*See also* EC.04.01.03, EP 1.)

EP 13: The [organization] conducts annual environmental tours in nonpatient care areas to

evaluate the effectiveness of previously implemented activities intended to minimize or eliminate risks in the environment. (*See also* EC.04.01.03, EP 1.)

STANDARD EC.04.01.05

The [organization] improves its environment of care.

Environmental tours or rounds are among the most useful tools for assessing infection risks and evaluating the use of infection prevention practices in a variety of health care settings. Tours should be done by a multidisciplinary team, performed on a set schedule, and documented using a standardized form. The team should consist of infection prevention and control personnel, supervisory and nonsupervisory personnel from the area being surveyed, housekeeping staff, facilities maintenance staff, safety personnel, and staff from other areas as needed.

To demonstrate compliance with this standard, the findings and recommendations for corrective measures or performance improvement, as revealed by the environmental tours or other assessment methods, should be documented. They should be sent to the multidisciplinary team members and those who are able to effect the needed corrections or desired improvements. There should also be evidence that the corrections and improvements were effectively implemented. (As previously mentioned, sample environmental rounds forms can be found in the "CD Tools" section of this chapter.)

TIP: An infection preventionist should monitor and document daily the negative airflow in airborne infection isolation rooms and the positive airflow in protective environment rooms, especially when patients are in these rooms, as recommended by the CDC.[1]

SUMMARY

The health care environment can serve as a source of pathogenic organisms. To ensure a safe environment, a health care organization must assess the role that the environment plays in potential infection risks. Based on the risk assessment, the organization must identify and implement measures that will reduce the risk of transmission or acquisition of organisms to patients, staff, or visitors from environmental sources. In addition, the organization must monitor compliance with these measures. This chapter discusses a variety of measures that organizations can use to provide a safe health care environment and monitor the effectiveness of infection prevention activities.

FURTHER RESOURCES

The following sections provide further information on this topic and can serve as a valuable reference in implementing measures to ensure a safe health care environment.

CD Tools

Tool 8-1: Infection Control Risk Assessment Matrix of Precautions for Construction and Renovation—St. Francis Hospital

Tool 8-2: Infection Control Construction Permit—St. Francis Hospital

Tool 8-3: San Ramon Regional Medical Center, Construction and Renovation: Infection Control Checklist

Tool 8-4: Infection Control Construction Rounds Compliance Monitor—Genesis HealthCare System

Tool 8-5: Environmental Rounds, Infection Control—Skaggs Regional Medical Center

Tool 8-6: University Medical Center Hospital Renovation and New Construction Projects
    a.   Infection Control Risk Assessment (ICRA)
    b.   Infection Control Permit
    c.   Construction Rounds
    d.   Standard Policy and Procedure

Tool 8-7: University of Louisville Hospital—Daily Monitoring: ILSM - ICRA Precautions

Tool 8-8: A Risk-rating Tool for Hospital Warm Water Systems

Tool 8-9: West Virginia University Hospitals—Environmental Rounds, Infection Control

Tool 8-10: Environmental Tour Checklist—Sky Ridge Medical Center

Tool 8-11: Facility Guidelines and Expectations for Contractors—University of New Mexico Hospitals

Tool 8-12: Infection Control and Safety Construction Compliance Monitor—Cooley Dickenson Hospital

Tool 8-13: Meriter IC Program Construction Signs—Meriter Hospital, Inc.

Tool 8-14: Construction Risk Assessment and Management Plan—Meriter Hospital, Inc.

Tool 8-15: IC Physician Office/Clinic Checklist—McKay-Dee Hospital Center

Tool 8-16: IC Hospital Unit Checklist—McKay-Dee Hospital Center

Tool 8-17: IC OR Checklist—McKay-Dee Hospital Center

Web Sites

- American Society for Healthcare Engineering of the American Hospital Association: http://www.ashe.org.
- American Society for Heating, Refrigeration, and Air Conditioning Engineers: http://www.ashrae.org.
- Association for the Advancement of Medical Instrumentation: http://www.aami.org. Standards for dialysis water quality, storage, and distribution and standards for disinfection and sterilization in health care settings.
- Association of periOperative Registered Nurses: http://www.aorn.org. Standards for operating rooms and cleaning, disinfection, and sterilization of equipment.
- Centers for Disease Control and Prevention: *Infection Control in Healthcare Settings.* http://www.cdc.gov/ncidod/dhqp/index.html.
- Centers for Disease Control and Prevention: *Legionellosis Resource Site.* http://www.cdc.gov/legionella/index.htm.
- FDA Medical Devices Web site. http://www.fda.gov/MedicalDevices/DeviceRegulationandGuidance/ReprocessingofSingle-UseDevices/ucm121544.htm#guidances. Contains a variety of documents on reprocessing single-use devices.
- Rutala W.: *Disinfection and Sterilization.* http://disinfectionandsterilization.org. Guidelines and resources on cleaning, disinfection, and sterilization in health care settings.
- Special Pathogens Laboratory: http://www.legionella.org/. Publications and guidelines related to Legionella.

Additional Readings

- American Institute of Architects (AIA): *Guidelines for Design and Construction of Hospitals and Health Care Facilities*. Washington, DC: AIA, 2006. Available at http://www.aia.org/index.htm.

- Association for Professionals in Infection Control and Epidemiology (APIC): *APIC Text of Infection Control and Epidemiology*, 3rd ed. Washington, DC: APIC, 2009. Available at http://www.apic.org. The following *APIC Text* chapters are applicable to the topics in this chapter:
  — Chapter 55: "Central Services"
  — Chapter 56: "Physician Office"
  — Chapter 57: "Reprocessing Single-Use Devices"
  — Chapter 101: "Laundry, Patient Linens, Textiles, and Uniforms"
  — Chapter 102: "Waste Management"
  — Chapter 103: "Maintenance and Engineering"
  — Chapter 104: "Heating, Ventilation, and Air Conditioning"
  — Chapter 105: "Water Systems Issues and Prevention of Waterborne Infectious Diseases in Healthcare Facilities"
  — Chapter 106: "Construction and Renovation"

- The Joint Commission: *Environment of Care Handbook*, 3rd ed. Oakbrook Terrace, IL: Joint Commission Resources, 2009.

- The Joint Commission: *Planning, Design, and Construction of Health Care Facilities*, 2nd ed. Oakbrook Terrace, IL: Joint Commission Resources, 2009.

REFERENCES

1. Sehulster L.M., et al.: *HICPAC Guidelines for Environmental Control in Health-Care Facilities. Recommendations from CDC and the Healthcare Infection Control Practices Advisory Committee (HICPAC)*. Centers for Disease Control and Prevention, 2003. http://www.cdc.gov/ncidod/dhqp/gl_environinfection.html (accessed May 31, 2009).

2. Johnston C.P., et al.: Outbreak management and implications of a nosocomial norovirus outbreak. *Clin Infect Dis* 45:534–540, 2007.

3. Occupational Safety and Health Administration: *Standard 29 CFR 1910.1030: Bloodborne Pathogens*. http://www.osha.gov/pls/oshaweb/searchresults.category?p_text=bloodborne%20pathogens&p_title=&p_status=CURRENT (accessed Jul. 13, 2009).

4. U.S. Environmental Protection Agency: *Medical Waste Frequent Questions*. http://www.epa.gov/osw/nonhaz/industrial/medical/mwfaqs.htm (accessed Jul. 13, 2009).

5. Association of periOperative Registered Nurses: *Perioperative Standards and Recommended Practices*. 2009. http://www.aorn.org/PracticeResources/AORNStandardsAndRecommendedPractices/ (accessed Jul. 23, 2009).

6. Association for the Advancement of Medical Instrumentation (AAMI): *ANSI/AAMI ST79:2006 and ANSI/AAMI ST79/A1 2008. Comprehensive Guide to Steam Sterilization and Sterilization Assurance in Health Care Facilities*. Arlington, VA: AAMI, 2008.

7. Centers for Disease Control and Prevention: *Guidelines for Disinfection and Sterilization in Healthcare Facilities*. 2008. http://www.cdc.gov/ncidod/dhqp/sterile.html (accessed Jul. 14, 2009).

8. Food and Drug Administration (FDA): *Enforcement Priorities for Single-Use Devices Reprocessed by Third Parties and Hospitals*. 2000. http://www.fda.gov/MedicalDevices/DeviceRegulationandGuidance/GuidanceDocuments/ucm107164.htm (accessed Jul. 14, 2009).

9. Pegues D.A., et al.: Anaphylactoid reactions associated with reuse of hollow-fiber hemodialyzers and ACE inhibitors. *Kidney Int* 42:1232–1237, 1992.

10. Gordon S.M., et al.: Epidemic hypotension in a dialysis center caused by sodium azide. *Kidney Int* 37:110–115, 1990.

11. Carmichael W.W., et al.: Human fatalities from Cyanobacteria: Chemical and biological evidence for cyanotoxins. *Environ Health Perspect* 109, 2001. http://ehpnet1.niehs.nih.gov/docs/2001/109p663-668carmichael/abstract.html (accessed Jul. 14, 2009).

12. Association for the Advancement of Medical Instrumentation (AAMI): *DialysisStandards Collection*. Arlington, VA: AAMI, 2007. Available at http://www.aami.org/publications/standards/dialysis.html.

13. American Institute of Architects (AIA): *Guidelines for Design and Construction of Hospitals and Health Care Facilities*. Washington, DC: AIA, 2001.

14. Centers for Disease Control and Prevention: HICPAC guidelines for preventing health-care–associated pneumonia, 2003. *MMWR Recomm Rep* 53, 2004. http://www.cdc.gov/mmwr/preview/mmwrhtml/rr5303a1.htm (accessed Jul. 14, 2009).

15. Centers for Disease Control and Prevention: HICPAC guidelines for preventing the transmission of mycobacterium tuberculosis in health-care settings, 2005. *MMWR Recomm Rep* 54, 2005. http://www.cdc.gov/mmwr/preview/mmwrhtml/rr5417a1.htm?s_cid=rr5417a1_e (accessed Jul. 14, 2009).

16. American Society for Heating, Refrigeration, and Air Conditioning Engineers (ASHRAE): Standard 62.1-2004—Ventilation for Acceptable Indoor Air Quality (ANSI Approved). Atlanta: ASHRAE, 2004.

Chapter 9

Occupational Health Issues

Tammy S. Lundstrom, M.D., J.D.; and Susan Sebazco, R.N., B.S., C.I.C.

Preventing infection transmission from health care workers to patients and from patients to health care workers is a key goal of an occupational health program. Each organization should have such a program and design it to create and maintain an environment that is as safe as possible for workers and the persons to whom they provide care.

The relationship of an infection prevention and control (IPC) program to an organization's occupational health program will vary, depending on the organization's patient population, the services offered, and the prevalence of diseases in the surrounding community. Depending on the setting, elements of an occupational health program that relate to infection prevention and control can include the following:

- Surveillance and assessments
- Immunizations
- Education
- Postexposure management
- Exposure prevention and control

The Joint Commission "Infection Prevention and Control" (IC) standards delineate what organizations must do to meet the requirements of providing a safe work environment for health care personnel. Specifically, Standard IC.02.03.01 and Standard IC.02.04.01 address this issue. This chapter takes a closer look at these two standards and discusses ways for organizations to ensure compliance.

STANDARD IC.02.03.01

The [organization] works to prevent the transmission of infectious disease among patients, licensed independent practitioners, and staff.

EXPLORING IC.02.03.01

Standard IC.02.03.01 requires organizations to engage in activities that prevent the transmission of infectious disease among patients and health care workers. The following discussion describes some of the activities that infection preventionists can use to meet this standard, as it relates to occupational health.

IC.02.03.01, EP 1: The [organization] makes screening for exposure and/or immunity to infectious disease available to licensed independent practitioners and staff who may come in contact with infections at the workplace.

The recent literature is replete with descriptions of outbreaks of vaccine-preventable diseases—including measles,[1,2] pertussis,[3,4] and mumps[5–7] among others—in which health care workers played a role in transmission. In addition to these diseases, the 2003 severe acute respiratory syndrome (SARS) outbreak highlighted the role that health care workers can play in transmitting diseases and emphasized the need to screen and furlough exposed personnel in order to halt further nosocomial transmission.[8]

The Joint Commission standards are designed to help prevent transmission of vaccine-preventable diseases from health care workers to patients and vice versa. Prevention of infection transmission requires proactive screening for exposure and immunity in order to assess facility transmission risks. According to The Joint Commission Web site (http://www.jointcommission.org/standards/FAQs/), health screenings are a requirement for employees to whom the "Human Resources" (HR) standards apply. Screenings must be made available to nonemployed physicians and other licensed independent practitioners; however, each organization may decide whether these screenings should be mandatory. When making this decision, organizations should also take into consideration any local or state requirements to which they are bound.

TIP: *Prevention of infection transmission between health care workers and patients requires proactive screening for exposure and immunity in order to assess facility transmission risks.*

If the status of a health care worker would put patients at risk of acquiring communicable diseases, the organization must provide or refer the worker to treatment, prophylaxis, counseling, or immunization to mitigate the risk. These activities could apply to diseases such as tuberculosis (TB), hepatitis B, varicella, pertussis, mumps, rubella, measles, and influenza.

To further prevent the transmission of specific infectious diseases, an organization should document evidence of health care worker immunity, such as immunity to varicella, measles, mumps, and rubella. Most organizations take steps to ensure immunity to these diseases as conditions of employment. In other words, if, upon testing, an employee is nonimmune, he or she is immunized as a condition of employment in the organization, unless contraindications to immunization exist. Most organizations also allow exemptions for religious reasons.

TIP: *In order to accomplish the objectives of Standard IC.02.03.01, it is important that the leaders of the IPC program maintain a close working relationship with both the human resources department and the occupational medicine department. These two departments should set the policies that determine what health screening and laboratory studies will be performed in both newly hired and current health care personnel. In addition, the two departments need to work together to develop policies related to health care worker furlough and return to work in relation to potentially exposed and ill workers.*

For staff working with specific populations, such as neonates or children, the organization may wish to focus on screens and immunizations for staff to prevent infections that could jeopardize the patients. For example, because infants younger than 6 months old cannot receive influenza vaccination, a major prevention strategy for this age group is to immunize contacts, including families and health care workers.[9]

To ensure compliance with this element of performance (EP), the infection preventionist should be familiar with the screening and immunization policies for the organization and should periodically compare them to current recommendations issued by outside entities, such as the Centers for Disease Control and Prevention's (CDC's) Advisory Committee on Immunization Practices (ACIP)[10] as well as other agencies. (*See* Sidebar 9-1 on page 109.)

IC.02.03.01, EP 2: When licensed independent practitioners or staff have, or are suspected of having, an infectious disease that puts others at risk, the [organization] provides them with or refers them for assessment, testing, immunization, prophylaxis/treatment, or counseling.

A recent example highlighting the necessity for assessment, testing, immunization, treatment, and counseling of potentially infected staff is the novel H1N1 influenza A pandemic that began in 2009. In this case, because the seasonal influenza vaccine did not provide adequate protection, it was initially crucial to identify health care workers who had been exposed to un-isolated cases in order to provide them with antiviral prophylaxis. The very short incubation period of this influenza (1–4 days) presented a challenge and reinforced the need to have rapid and reliable communication channels between the infection prevention and control team, unit management, and occupational health.

In cases such as the H1N1 influenza A pandemic, health care organizations may consider conducting twice-daily "touch base" conference calls or meetings to be assured that all departments are working together to achieve patient and staff safety. In addition, organizations need to have a means to identify workers who may have been exposed in the community or who develop symptoms in order to treat them, provide them prophylaxis, and furlough them. This is necessary to prevent further nosocomial spread. An infection preventionist should participate in the policy development and communication in these situations, even though the occupational health service will generally assume coordination and oversight responsibilities.

Sidebar 9-1: Other Agencies' Standards

In addition to The Joint Commission, other agencies, such as the Occupational Safety and Health Administration (OSHA) and state occupational health agencies, generate regulations related to employee safety and infection transmission risk. For example, OSHA, through the Bloodborne Pathogens Standard, requires that health care workers who will have potential exposure to blood or other potentially infectious material be offered the vaccination series against hepatitis B virus prior to engaging in activities to which they could be exposed.[11] OSHA requires those who decline the vaccine to sign a declination form.[11] OSHA's Web site provides health care–wide modules and e-tools that address bloodborne pathogens and TB. The e-tools outline potential hazards addressed in the standards relative to health care settings and include model plans and programs and direct links to enforcement procedures.[12]

Like OSHA, the Federal Needlestick Safety and Prevention Act[13] requires that frontline health care workers participate in the selection of devices with engineered sharps safety protection and that all safety devices available be utilized unless there is a patient or employee safety issue identified with the use of the device.

The Centers for Disease Control and Prevention (CDC) also offers a very comprehensive prevention workbook that includes tools and worksheets to assist those in occupational medicine and infection prevention in managing their entire sharps safety program.[14] In addition, the CDC provides helpful resources on its Web site for a comprehensive tuberculosis program.[15] Here one can find not only guidelines but fact sheets and educational materials, including slide sets that can help a program meet regulatory and accreditation requirements.

One of the roles of an infection preventionist is to be familiar with the latest evidence-based guidelines and requirements, such as those from OSHA, in order to ensure that the program remains in compliance.[16] (See the Web sites listed in the "Further Resources" section at the end of this chapter.)

TIP: *An IPC program's annual risk assessment should include a review of occupational health experiences to identify any trends related to infection that should be addressed in the plan. The annual review may include examination of occupational exposure data, a sharps injury log, data on occupationally acquired or transmitted diseases, and information about community-acquired infections identified in health care workers. Sample risk assessment plans that show how this may be accomplished are included in Chapter 4.*

IC.02.03.01, EP 3: When licensed independent practitioners or staff have been occupationally exposed to an infectious disease, the [organization] provides them with or refers them for assessment, testing, immunization, prophylaxis/treatment, or counseling.

IC.02.03.01, EP 3, is designed to ensure that health care workers who are placed at risk in the work environment, by potential or real exposure to an infectious disease, are pro-vided with support to quickly assess the extent and severity of the exposure and to determine how to manage it.

TIP: *A potential health care worker exposure of which organizations should be aware is pertussis exposure. This type of exposure has become more commonplace. When a tetanus toxoid, reduced diphtheria toxoid, and acellular pertussis vaccine (Tdap), formulated for use in adults, was licensed in the United States in 2005, many organizations adjusted their immunization programs to include this vaccine for health care workers. Adjustments were also made for vaccines that are offered to certain patient populations, such as administering Tdap in place of tetanus toxoid boosters in the emergency department and offering Tdap to mothers postdelivery and prior to discharge.[17] For those facilities where experts in exposure management are not available on site, a National Clinician's Post-Exposure Prophylaxis Hotline (PEP-Line) is available 24/7 at 888/448-4911.*

Consider this example: A health care worker sustains a sharps injury from a patient known to have a bloodborne pathogen. In this case, because time is of the essence (especially if the pathogen is HIV), many facilities would utilize their emer-gency department after hours and have rapid triage policies to ensure that exposed health care workers are seen expeditiously.

Other facilities would have clinical staff on call who could respond immediately and provide phone counseling and assessment, as well as order treatment through the use of protocols and algorithms.

To promptly address exposure risks, health care workers should be aware of signs, symptoms, and potential exposures that should prompt a call to occupational health or infection prevention and control.[18] It is also important for those who are counseling exposed health care workers to be clear about work restrictions and return-to-work policies, required documentation, communication with supervisors of the exposed staff member, and any reports that should be sent to leadership.

When a health care worker is exposed to an infectious disease, it is important to be able to easily access his or her immunization records to determine what precautions or work restrictions are necessary. For this reason, an organization should maintain immunization and immune status records in a readily retrievable database.

IC.02.03.01, EP 4: When patients have been exposed to an infectious disease, the [organization] provides them with or refers them for assessment, testing, immunization, prophylaxis/treatment, or counseling.

Sometimes, patients are exposed to infectious diseases in health care settings in spite of systems and practices to prevent such exposures. It is an organization's responsibility to provide appropriate care to a patient after any exposure that may place the patient, or subsequently his or her family or visitors, at risk of acquiring an infectious disease.

Postexposure management can include treatment, prophylaxis, counseling, and vaccination, as appropriate. Not only is addressing exposure required when patients are exposed to diseases such as TB, hepatitis B or C, varicella, pertussis, mumps, rubella, measles, and influenza, but it is also required when a whole host of other transmissible infectious diseases are present for which no vaccination exists, such as blood and body fluid exposures, meningococcal meningitis, scabies, or emerging pathogens such as SARS or novel H1N1 influenza.

TIP: *It is an organization's responsibility to provide appropriate care to a patient after any exposure that may place the patient, or subsequently his or her family or visitors, at risk of acquiring an infectious disease.*

An infection preventionist should participate in developing and reviewing the protocols for postexposure management for health care workers and patients. An infection preventionist should also ensure, with occupational health, that those who will assess exposed staff and patients have current knowledge about postexposure management and access to vaccines or other medications for prophylaxis.

To help with compliance efforts, organizations should consider developing a script for use in counseling staff and patients to ensure that standard information is conveyed, laws are followed, and staff and patients are aware of the risks from the exposure and the steps that are recommended to prevent infections, when possible. For either staff or patients, postexposure management should include consideration of family members and visitors who may have been or could be at risk for secondary exposure.

An important issue for health care organizations is the accessibility to evaluation and care by both staff and patients, whether such evaluation and care is administered during occupational health office hours or after hours in the emergency department or in a central location off site from the organization. When a patient needs to be followed, the patient's primary care physician should be informed and involved in the evaluation and care.

EXPLORING IC.02.04.01

Standard IC.02.04.01 requires organizations to offer vaccination against influenza to licensed independent practitioners and staff. The following sections look at each of the EPs associated with this standard.

> ### STANDARD IC.02.04.01
> The [organization] offers vaccination against influenza to licensed independent practitioners and staff.

IC.02.04.01, EP 1: The [organization] establishes an annual influenza vaccination program that is offered to licensed independent practitioners and staff.

Annual vaccination for influenza is commonly acknowledged as a way to preserve both staff and patient safety. For example, the CDC's ACIP for many years has recommended annual influenza vaccination of health care workers as a patient safety measure to prevent the transmission of influenza from health care workers to others.[19] Likewise, many professional societies and organizations, including the Society for Healthcare Epidemiology of America (SHEA),[20] the Association for Professionals in Infection Control and Epidemiology (APIC),[21] the Infectious Diseases Society of America (IDSA),[22] and the National Foundation for Infectious Diseases (NFID)[23] promote annual vaccination of health care workers as a means to improve patient safety. Despite such recommendations, as of the 2005–2006 seasons, only 42% of health care workers reported having received the influenza vaccination in the National Health Interview Survey (NHIS).[24]

Annual influenza vaccination of health care workers may be the most challenging of the occupational health–related standards, because of the scope and time frame involved in the vaccinations. Consider that activities such as annual TB evaluations can be spread throughout the year, but influenza season mandates mass vaccinations over a shorter time frame.

To comply with IC.02.04.01, EP 1, an organization must demonstrate that it has an annual influenza vaccination program that includes licensed independent practitioners and staff. Organizations can demonstrate this by discussing the annual immunization program and the vaccination acceptance rates in the annual IPC plan, as discussed in Chapter 4.

An infection preventionist has a pivotal role in providing guidance and assistance to the occupational health service and organization leadership to develop and establish a proactive immunization program. This may involve providing literature, developing polices, participating in education, and analyzing data with the occupational health service.

IC.02.04.01, EP 2: The [organization] educates licensed independent practitioners and staff about, at a minimum, the influenza vaccine; non-vaccine control and prevention measures; and the diagnosis, transmission, and impact of influenza.

Infection preventionists should join with educators and occupational health staff in their organization to provide education to health care workers on multiple aspects of influenza, including the following:

- Diagnosis
- Transmission
- Disease impact on patients, health care workers, and the community
- Influenza prevention measures
- Dispelling of myths associated with influenza. This may be the most challenging aspect of the educational effort.

Many options and tools are available for education, including posters, brochures, fact sheets, videos, and Webcasts and podcasts from the CDC, state health departments, the World Health Organization, and many other professional organizations (*see* the "Further Resources" section at the end of this chapter). In addition to external resources, internal resources, such as Web-based and DVD programs, can also be developed. One-on-one education during rounds on units and in departments throughout the organization can also be effective.

To demonstrate compliance with IC.02.04.01, EP 2, organizations can incorporate a section on educational programs provided to health care workers within the organization's IPC plan.

If compliance is a problem in an organization, an infection preventionist and others may wish to perform a survey or convene a focus group of key staff to determine the barriers to acceptance of the vaccine. The information gained from these activities can be incorporated into future educational efforts or approaches to vaccine administration.

TIP: *Computer screen savers can be developed that include information on influenza vaccination (as well as other pertinent infection prevention topics).*

IC.02.04.01, EP 3: The [organization] provides influenza vaccination at sites accessible to licensed independent practitioners and staff.

One barrier to immunization can be the lack of accessibility to the influenza vaccine. This may occur when vaccine administration is off site from the primary work setting; the vaccine is only administered during occupational health office hours, which do not include evening or weekend hours; or the vaccine administration time period is limited to certain months of the year.

One method for complying with IC.02.04.01, EP 3, is to provide the influenza vaccine at the point of care, such as by taking a cart with the vaccine and related supplies to clinical and support units. This eliminates the need for health care workers to come to the occupational health department to receive the vaccine.

Another approach is to provide the vaccine to a designated staff member on each unit, who can then administer the vaccine to coworkers and others. Departmental and other meetings held during the influenza season can also be used as to vaccinate multiple staff in one convenient setting. Some organizations have expanded the weeks or months for administering the vaccine to improve vaccination rates.

TIP: *Some organizations take advantage of the need to annually vaccinate health care workers for influenza as a means to test their mass vaccination capabilities. They choose a one- to two-day time period for vaccinating as many staff as possible, thus also testing their emergency management system's ability to provide mass vaccination or prophylaxis in the event of a pandemic or bioterrorism event.*[25]

IC.02.04.01, EP 4: The [organization] annually evaluates vaccination rates and the reasons given for declining the influenza vaccination.

The Joint Commission requires that an organization evaluate its influenza vaccination program. This may involve calculating vaccination rates, surveying health care workers about why they do not get vaccinated, and working to improve vaccination rates. (*See* Figure 9-1 on page 113.) To meet this requirement, most organizations calculate rates of vaccine administration either overall for the organization or by various clinical or support units. Some analyze gender, profession, work shift, work setting, and other variables to get a precise picture of where there is an opportunity for improvement. It is important to note that these data may not be exact because some health care workers get their immunizations elsewhere. Information collected can then be used to target educational programs to improve vaccination acceptance.

One option afforded organizations is the use of a declination form for those who are eligible for but refuse the vaccine or explain that they have received the vaccine elsewhere. Many health care workers, especially physicians, work at other facilities and may have been immunized there, by their personal physician, or at another community site. Controversy exists over whether a declination form should be implemented for those refusing vaccination. (*See* Tool 9-1 in the "CD Tools" section for a sample declination form.)

IC.02.04.01, EP 5: The [organization] takes steps to increase influenza vaccination rates.

To satisfy IC.02.04.01, EP 5, an organization can implement a quality improvement program designed to improve influenza vaccination rates. The program can use the results from health care worker surveys, focus groups, or other information sources to identify why workers do not get vaccinated; the program can develop action plans to improve vaccination rates. An infection preventionist can provide valuable expertise in the design and implementation of these activities. The actions taken to improve compliance, and the effectiveness of these interventions, can be documented in an organization's IPC plan and program evaluation. (*See* Sidebar 9-2 on page 114.)

To help improve vaccination rates, some facilities have mandated annual influenza vaccination as a condition of employment. For example, The Barnes Jewish, Christian (BJC) Health Care System initiated such a program during the 2008–2009 influenza season and achieved a compliance rate of 99.97%. The success of this approach was dependent on extensive and all-inclusive planning, as well as many town hall meetings that provided health care workers with an opportunity to ask questions and have their concerns addressed.[26]

Figure 9-1. Health Care Worker Influenza Vaccination Survey

1. I received a flu shot in the time period from September 1, 20–, to March 1, 20–.

   ☐ Yes, I received my flu shot at _____Hospital [Stop here]

   ☐ Yes, I received my flu shot at my doctor's office [Stop here]

   ☐ Yes, I received my flu shot at another location [Stop here]

   ☐ No, I did not receive a flu shot during this flu season [GO ON TO ADDITIONAL QUESTIONS]

2. I did not receive a flu shot during this flu season because: (Check all that apply)

   ☐ I am concerned I will get the flu from the shot

   ☐ I am concerned I will have a reaction to the flu shot

   ☐ I always get sick after the flu shot

   ☐ I am afraid of shots

   ☐ I didn't have time

   ☐ Getting the vaccine was not convenient

   ☐ I never get the flu

   ☐ I am allergic to eggs

   ☐ My doctor advised against it

   ☐ Immunization is against my religion

   ☐ Other_____

3. If I could be protected from the flu without having to get a shot, I would do it.

   ☐ Yes

   ☐ No

This is a sample survey designed to identify why health care workers do not get immunized. This tool can be distributed either via paper or electronically.

Source: Susan Sebazco, R.N., B.S., C.I.C.

TIP: *In 2008, Joint Commission Resources hosted its first Flu Vaccination Challenge blog. Registered participants used this online community to share experiences, thoughts, comments, resources, and best practices relative to increasing flu vaccination rates among health care workers. (A summary of this blog is provided in Tool 9-2 in the "CD Tools" section.)*

Sidebar 9-2: Key Activities to Help Meet the Occupational Health–Related Standards

- Include communicable diseases and occupational health issues in your annual facility risk assessment (*see* Chapter 4).
- List approaches to compliance with occupational health–related standards in the annual infection prevention and control plan.
- Establish lines of communication and develop a close working relationship with the occupational health service and human resources department.
- Proactively develop, implement, and ensure compliance with postexposure protocols for common communicable diseases for staff, nonemployed physicians, and other licensed independent practitioners, as well as patients. Work in concert with occupational health services.
- Define in policy or procedure who is responsible for each aspect of a communicable diseases exposure investigation. (For example, an organization may designate a clinical manager to be responsible for developing an employee and patient exposure list, with input from infection prevention and control.)
- Educate health care workers about what signs, symptoms, and potential exposures should prompt a call to occupational health or infection prevention and control.
- Provide an annual influenza vaccination program that is offered to licensed independent practitioners and staff, includes education regarding vaccination benefits for staff and patients, is accessible, and is evaluated for effectiveness.

SUMMARY

This chapter provides a brief overview of the infection control standards that relate to occupational health. It discusses the importance of screening and vaccinating health care workers for specific infectious diseases as well as responding to the needs of potentially and actually infected staff and patients. Specifically, the chapter focuses on providing vaccinations to prevent the spread of influenza, requiring organizations to educate staff members about the importance of the vaccinations, monitor the vaccination rate, and improve that rate, where warranted.

FURTHER RESOURCES

The following sections provide further information on this topic and can serve as a valuable reference in preserving occupational health and safety.

CD Tools

Tool 9-1: Declination Form for Influenza Vaccination

Tool 9-2: Effective Approaches for Increasing Vaccination Rates

Tool 9-3: Suggested Components for Compliance with Standard IC.02.02.01 and Standard IC.02.04.01

Additional Readings
The American Journal of Medicine
- Schaffner W., ed.: Expanding the influenza vaccination season: A new paradigm for increasing immunization rates. *Am J Med* 121(Suppl. 2):LS1–S2, Jul. 2008.

Association for Professionals in Infection Control and Epidemiology (APIC): http://www.apic.org
- Position papers:
  — APIC Position on Influenza Immunization of Healthcare Personnel
  — Mandatory Vaccination of Healthcare Workers
  — Toolkit for ICPs to Increase Health Care Worker Influenza Immunization

Centers for Disease Control and Prevention: http://www.cdc.gov
- Healthcare workers occupational health and other infection prevention guidelines: http://www.cdc.gov/ncidod/dhqp/guidelines.html.

- Influenza: http://www.cdc.gov/flu.
- Tuberculosis in health care settings: http://www.cdc.gov/ncidod/dhqp/id_tb.html.
- Advisory Committee on Immunization Practices (ACIP) http://www.cdc.gov/vaccines/recs/ACIP/default.htm. ACIP Provisional Recommendations for Measles-Mumps-Rubella (MMR) "Evidence of Immunity" Requirements for Healthcare Personnel Source: Centers for Disease Control and Prevention, August 28, 2009

Joint Commission Resources: http://www.jcrinc.com

- Flu Vaccine Challenge: http://www.jcrinc.com/FLUChallenge.

National Foundation for Infectious Diseases: http://www.nfid.org

- Annual flu immunization campaigns and links to additional information: http://www.nfid.org/influenza.

Occupational Safety and Health Administration: http://www.osha.gov

- Health care–wide hazards: http://www.osha.gov/SLTC/etools/hospital/hazards/sharps/sharps.html.

Society for Healthcare Epidemiology of America (SHEA): http://www.shea-online.org

- *SHEA Position Paper: Influenza Vaccination of Healthcare Workers and Vaccine Allocation for Healthcare Workers During Vaccine Shortages*: http://www.shea-online.org/Assets/files/HCW_Flu_Position_Paper_FINAL_9-28.pdf.

World Health Organization

- Influenza: http://www.who.int/csr/disease/influenza/en

REFERENCES

1. Update measles—United States, January–July 2008. *MMWR Morb Mortal Wkly Rep* 57:893–896, 2008.
2. Outbreak of measles—San Diego, California, January–February 2008. *MMWR Morb Mortal Wkly Rep* 57:203–206, 2008.
3. Use of mass Tdap vaccination to control an outbreak of pertussis in a high school—Cook County Illinois, September 2006–January 2007. *MMWR Morb Mortal Wkly Rep* 57:796–799, 2008.
4. Hospital acquired Pertussis among newborns—Texas, 2004. *MMWR Morb Mortal Wkly Rep* 57:600–603, 2008.
5. Update: Multistate outbreak of mumps—United States, January 1–May 2, 2006. *MMWR Morb Mortal Wkly Rep* 55:559–563, 2006.
6. Exposure to mumps during air travel—United States, April 2006. *MMWR Morb Mortal Wkly Rep* 55:401–402, 2006.
7. Mumps epidemic—Iowa, 2006. *MMWR Morb Mortal Wkly Rep* 55:366–368, 2006.
8. Centers for Disease Control and Prevention: Preparedness and response in healthcare facilities. Supplement C in *Severe Acute Respiratory Syndrome, Public Health Guidance for Community-level Preparedness with Response to SARS (Version 2)*. May 3, 2005. http://www.cdc.gov/ncidod/sars/guidance/C/index.htm (accessed Oct. 9, 2009).
9. Centers for Disease Control and Prevention: *Children Aged 6–23 Months and Caregivers of Children Younger Than 6 Months Encouraged to Receive Influenza Vaccination*, Dec. 4, 2003. http://www.cdc.gov/media/archives.htm (accessed Jun. 25, 2009).
10. Centers for Disease Control and Prevention. Use of Influenza A (H1N1) 2009 Monovalent Vaccine. Recommendations of the Advisory Committee on Immunization Practices (ACIP), 2009. *MMWR Recomm Rep*, 58(No. RR-10):1–8, 2009.
11. Occupational Safety and Health Administration: Occupational exposure to bloodborne pathogens: Needlesticks and other sharps injuries. *Final Rule 29 CFR Part 1910 Federal Register* 66:5318–5325, 2001.
12. Occupational Safety and Health Administration: *Needlestick/Sharps Injuries.* http://www.osha.gov/SLTC/etools/hospital/hazards/sharps/sharps.html (accessed Jun. 20, 2009).
13. Needlestick Safety and Prevention Act. Law 106430, Nov 6, 2000. 106th Congress of the United States of America. http://thomas.loc.gov (accessed Mar. 31, 2009).
14. Centers for Disease Control and Prevention: *Workbook for Designing, Implementing and Evaluating a Sharps Injury Prevention Program*, 2008. http://www.cdc.gov/sharpssafety/ (accessed May 1, 2009).
15. Centers for Disease Control and Prevention: *Tuberculosis (TB).* http://www.cdc.gov/tb/default.htm (accessed May 1, 2009).
16. Occupational Safety and Health Administration: *Home page.* http://www.osha.gov (accessed Jun. 20, 2009).
17. Centers for Disease Control and Prevention: Preventing tetanus, diphtheria, and pertussis among adults: Use of tetanus toxoid, reduced diphtheria toxoid and acellular pertussis vaccine. *MMWR Recomm Rep* 55(RR-17):1–33, 2006.
18. Centers for Disease Control and Prevention: Guidelines for infection control in healthcare personnel, 1998. *Am J Infect Control* 26:289–354, 1998.
19. Centers for Disease Control and Prevention: Prevention and control of influenza: Recommendations of the Advisory Committee on Immunization Practices, 2008. *MMWR Recomm Rep* 57(RR-7):1–60, 2008.
20. Talbot T., et al.: Position paper: Influenza vaccination of healthcare workers and vaccine allocation for healthcare workers during vaccine shortages. *Infect Control Hosp Epidemiol* 26:882–890, 2005.

21. Association for Professionals in Infection Control and Epidemiology: *Position Paper: Influenza Immunization of Healthcare Personnel.* http://www.apic.org/AM/Template.cfm?Section=Search&section=Position_Statements1&template=/CM/ContentDisplay.cfm&ContentFileID=11049 (accessed May 1, 2009).

22. Infectious Diseases Society of America: *Pandemic and Seasonal Influenza: Principles for U.S. Action,* 2007. http://www.idsociety.org/influenza.htm (accessed Oct. 9, 2009).

23. National Foundation for Infectious Diseases: *Call to Action: Influenza Immunization Among Health Care Personnel.* 2008. http://www.nfid.org/pdf/publications/fluhealthcarecta08.pdf (accessed Oct. 9, 2009).

24. Centers for Disease Control and Prevention: *Table 3. Influenza Vaccination Coverage Levels for the 2005–06, 2006–07, and 2007–08 Influenza Seasons, by Population Group—National Health Interview Survey (NHIS), United States, 2006, 2007, and 2008, and National Immunization Survey (NIS), 2006 and 2007.* http://www.cdc.gov/flu/professionals/acip/coveragelevels.htm#tab 3 (accessed May 31, 2009).

25. The Joint Commission: *Providing a Safer Environment for Health Care Personnel and Patients Through Influenza Vaccination: Strategies from Research and Practice,* 2009. http://www.jointcommission.org/PatientSafety/InfectionControl/flu_monograph.htm (accessed Jun. 26, 2009).

26. Personal communication between the author and Denise Murphy, R.N., M.P.A., C.I.C.

Chapter 10

Evaluating the Effectiveness of an Infection Prevention and Control Program

Candace Friedman, M.P.H., C.I.C.; and Susan Slavish, B.S.N., M.P.H., C.I.C.

The previous chapters in this book discuss how to allocate resources to an infection prevention and control (IPC) program; identify risk within the program; implement interventions to reduce the likelihood and spread of infections; respond to infectious disease emergencies; communicate about infection prevention and control efforts; address infection control within the, environment of care; and preserve occupational health and safety. All these activities are critical to a successful IPC program, and organizations must evaluate the success of the activities and make adjustments to enhance performance, as necessary. The evaluation process provides thoughtful review of each of these program components and gives direction to planning for the next year. This chapter discusses the topic of IPC program evaluation and provides tips and strategies on how to effectively evaluate the IPC program.

STANDARD IC.03.01.01

The organization evaluates the effectiveness of its infection prevention and control plan.

EVALUATING PROGRAM EFFECTIVENESS

Evaluating the effectiveness of infection prevention and control interventions helps identify which activities of the IPC program are successful and which need to be changed to improve outcomes. The Joint Commission addresses the concept of evaluation in Standard IC.03.01.01. This standard and its elements of performance (EPs) bring together the other "Infection Prevention and Control" (IC) standards into a step-by-step process that allows infection prevention and control staff to maintain a continuous cycle of improve-

ment. The steps in the cycle include identifying and prioritizing risks, developing and revising goals, implementing and evaluating interventions, sharing evaluation results organizationally, and making plan revisions. (*See* Figure 10-1 on page 118.) These activities, particularly the evaluation function, are similar to many of the methods used as a routine part of quality improvement efforts, such as the plan-do-check-act process, Six Sigma, and Toyota Lean.[1-4]

TIP: *Standard IC.03.01.01 and its EPs bring together the other IC standards into a step-by-step process that allows the infection prevention and control staff to maintain a continuous cycle of improvement.*

An effective evaluation helps determine the extent to which an IPC program is addressing its most important risks and meeting outlined goals and objectives. Questions to answer in the evaluation process include "Is the program working?" and "Are the desired results being achieved?" The following components should be considered as part of the evaluation process:

- The program's progress toward achieving its goals and objectives
- Whether objectives should be changed, added, or removed, and why
- The previous year's successes and failures

This information should then be used in the subsequent year's risk analysis process.

The evaluation process should be dynamic, collaborative, and organizationwide. It should evaluate risks that are facility specific, consider internal and external risks, and promote thoughtful examination of the use and results of infection prevention activities.

TIP: *An effective evaluation helps determine the extent to which an IPC program is addressing its most important risks and meeting outlined goals and objectives.*

EXPLORING IC.03.01.01

Standard IC.03.01.01 has six EPs that an oganization must address to demonstrate compliance. The following sections discuss these EPs.

IC.03.01.01, EP 1: The [organization] evaluates the effectiveness of its infection prevention and control plan annually and whenever risks significantly change.

IC.03.01.01, EP 1, requires a review of the IPC plan at least annually. As discussed in Chapter 4, such a review determines effectiveness, outlines activities that are still required,

and indicate other issues that should be incorporated into the next year's IPC plan.

Changes in practice or services or unexpected events may result in new activities performed during the year. Noting these changes in the annual evaluation can help infection prevention and control staff describe what actions were taken and whether they need to be incorporated into the IPC program in the following year. When the organization adds a significant new service, such as cardiovascular surgery or neonatal intensive care, or a new site of care, such as a home health agency, these changes affect the scope of the IPC program. The evaluation process must include a review of these changes.

IC.03.01.01, EP 2: The evaluation includes a review of the following: The infection prevention and control plan's prioritized risks.

As previously mentioned, an annual risk analysis will help identify any changes that need to be made to the IPC

Figure 10-1. Annual Infection Prevention and Control Program Evaluation Process

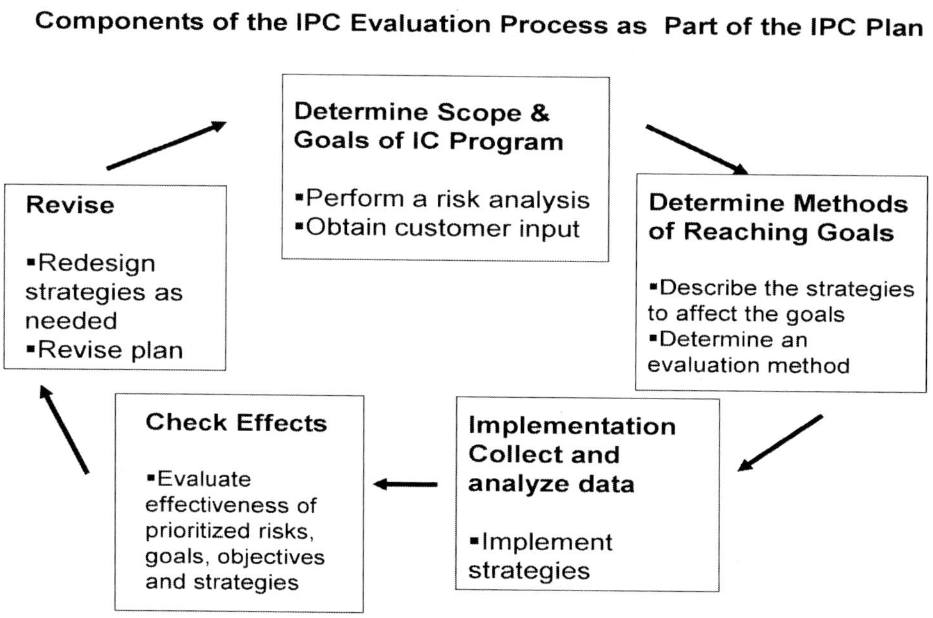

This figure illustrates the evaluation process as part of the infection prevention and control (IPC) program. IC, infection control.

Source: Candace Friedman, M.P.H., C.I.C.; and Susan Slavish, B.S.N., M.P.H., C.I.C.

program (*see* Chapter 4). The evaluation process reviews the success of the IPC program in addressing identified risks.

It may be helpful in designing the IPC program's goals and objectives to consider a tiered approach that could indicate achievements that are essential and those that would reflect exceptional accomplishments. For example, an evaluation process could identify that ventilator-associated infections have been reduced by 20% in the medical intensive care unit, or the evaluation could show that an organization has achieved a rate of zero central line–associated bloodstream infections (CLABSIs) for a three-month period. This type of evaluation provides the organization with a more precise description of the effectiveness of the infection prevention interventions.

IC.03.01.01, EP 3: The evaluation includes a review of the following: the infection prevention and control plan's goals.

The intent of IC.03.01.01, EP 3, is to guide the infection prevention and control team in purposefully reviewing the infection prevention and control goals and strategies for the year to determine whether goals were achieved or whether work needs to continue. As discussed in earlier chapters, the goals are developed to reflect the most significant risks, as determined in the risk assessment, and also those functions that are essential for maintaining an effective infection prevention program. The Joint Commission requires a minimum of five goals, including those related to prioritized risks; unprotected exposure to pathogens; transmission of infections during procedures or from medical equipment, devices, and supplies; and hand hygiene. (*See* Chapter 4.) The IPC program's goals and objectives should be aligned with the organization's goals and strategies and may need to be changed as those overarching goals and strategies are changed.

Many goals or objectives in one year might still be important in the next year. However, it is essential to reassess risks and review priorities for patients, staff, the environment of care, external threats, and other issues at least annually and to revise goals as appropriate.

IC.03.01.01, EP 4: The evaluation includes a review of the following: implementation of the infection prevention and control plan's activities.

IC.03.01.01, EP 4 addresses the evaluation of activities that were carried out to achieve the IPC program goals. When evaluating activities, it is important to document measurable achievements. For example, one could demonstrate the effectiveness of CLABSI-reducing interventions by showing a reduction in the rate of CLABSIs from the period before interventions were implemented to the period after interventions were implemented.

Within the evaluation process, it is important to determine what activities added value to the IPC program and contributed to improved patient safety and what activities should perhaps be revised or replaced by others that will better help to achieve the aims of the program. For example, if an education program for appropriate cleaning of the patient's environment has not resulted in improved practice, the infection preventionist and supervisor of environmental services may change the approach and include with the education program a supervised competency assessment, spot monitoring, a checklist for tasks, and regular feedback to staff.

IC.03.01.01, EP 5: Findings from the evaluation are communicated at least annually to the individuals or interdisciplinary group that manages the patient safety program.

It is important to communicate to leaders and others in the organization about problems or issues noted throughout the year as well as successes in meeting IPC program goals and objectives. Some things to consider when planning how to communicate about evaluation results include the following:

- Who are the primary audiences to receive the evaluation results? Consider individuals in leadership positions, including physician leaders, infection control committee members, and key staff, who can use the information to improve patient care.
- What kinds of information should be included in the evaluation report? The report can include all activities of the IPC program, investigations, summary data on health care–associated infections (HAIs), and goals for the next year.
- Where can that information be found, and how is it accessed? The information will be gathered from infection preventionist surveillance activities, employee health, and other services or departments performing monitoring activities related to the goals and objectives.
- How can the information be effectively reported? A report can be presented verbally, accompanied by a written report provided to a group such as within an

infection control or patient safety/quality improvement committee meeting, or it can be sent to appropriate individuals.

Each evaluation and reporting format will be somewhat different, depending on the needs and nature of the organization and its programs. (*See* Sidebar 10-1, below.)

One effective way to conduct and report a meaningful program evaluation is to develop a reporting template that incorporates the findings of the organizational infection prevention and control risk assessment. The template could include the following columns:

- Risks, goals, and objectives
- Strategies developed to achieve risk reduction
- Analysis methods and risk-reduction targets
- Individuals/departments responsible
- Progress toward achieving the objective or target

The report could be taken to the infection control and patient safety committees on a predetermined basis (for example, monthly, quarterly). Such a report could also be used to keep organizational and medical staff leadership informed on the organization's progress toward reducing infection risks.

Sidebar 10-1: Components of an Effective Evaluation Report

Because it is important to review activities and evaluate objectives, the evaluation report should consist of at least the following components:

1. A description of organizational changes that influenced the scope of the infection prevention and control (IPC) program

2. A review of each objective of the IPC program linked to the program's scope and goals. This should include activities performed to meet the goals and data that show how measurable objectives are being achieved. These data may be presented in a table or a graph and may come from a variety of sources, such as those that are presented in the institution's quality dashboard. Objectives that cannot be evaluated on the basis of data can be evaluated using qualitative methods, such as employee or patient feedback. These qualitative data can sometimes be converted to quantitative information. For example, if there is an objective to educate staff on a particular topic, a pre- and posteducation evaluation of knowledge about the topic can be performed and described, and rates can be calculated for posteducation test scores for all participants or for subtopics in the evaluation tool.

   Observation is another method for evaluating objectives. Observation results are often used to measure hand hygiene or isolation precautions practices. A hand hygiene observation surrogate may be the amount of hand hygiene product used. This can be measured by comparing the amount of product purchased and assigned to each area versus the amount used in the designated time period. This method does not provide specific information about variables such as the following: who used the product (staff, family, visitors); whether an adequate amount of product was used by each person; whether the product was used correctly; which professional groups used the product; and during which shifts the product was used. Hand hygiene observations can be reported as quantitative data by calculating the percentage of time hands are cleaned when there is an opportunity for hand hygiene or how often the technique for hand hygiene meets the criteria in the policy/procedure.

3. A summary of any important issue or activity that was not part of a specific objective. These issues or activities may become part of the next year's objectives. Examples may include an emergency that occurred during the time period, new construction activities, the investigation of practices at a new facility opened by the organization, or special assigned projects.

4. A summary of investigations performed during the year

5. A description of the challenges that occurred over the year and actions implemented. This information will influence planning for the coming year.

The written evaluation of the IPC program should be incorporated into the IPC plan and distributed to appropriate staff.

Another method for describing the findings of an annual evaluation is a summary report. An organization may already have an annual infection control committee or department report that can serve as the basis for the evaluation report. The evaluation can be performed collaboratively by individuals, a group of stakeholders, or a committee—for example, the infection control committee—and summarized in the existing report. (*See* Table 10-1 on page 122 and Tool 10-2 on the CD.)

TIP: *If an infection control committee exists, its members should receive a copy of the written evaluation. In addition, the chief executive officer, chief of staff, chief of nursing, patient safety leader, and other appropriate organization leaders and individuals should receive a copy.*

The most important aspect of evaluation reporting is ensuring that receivers interpret the data as the sender intended. Make sure the information provided in the evaluation report is appropriate for the individual(s) or group. There are several ways to ensure effective communication about IPC program evaluation, including the following[5]:

- Apply the seven *C*'s of effective communication: clear, correct, concise, cohesive, concrete, courteous, and complete.
- Include graphic aids to enhance the written presentation.
- Document all sources, using references as appropriate.

IC.03.01.01, EP 6: The [organization] uses the findings of its evaluation of the infection prevention and control plan when revising the plan.

As the IPC plan is evaluated, areas of necessary future work will be uncovered. These problems or issues should be incorporated into the annual risk analysis; the evaluation should state whether each issue should become an IPC program objective for the following year.

TIP: *Organizations must consider what decisions need to be made as a result of the evaluation. These might include changes to the risk assessment or priorities or changes in practice.*

COST EVALUATION

An area to consider during the evaluation process is the cost of infections and the value of the IPC program. Measuring the cost of HAIs is difficult, and the financial impact varies between different health care systems. However, there are areas on which to focus, such as length of stay, treatment costs, increased use of laboratory and other testing, and patient morbidity and mortality. In addition, there are investigation and control costs and potential legal liability.[6] One suggested strategy is to combine the institution's data on the reduction in HAI rates achieved through infection prevention and control efforts with estimates of benefit from well-designed studies in the health care literature, adjusting for the effect of inflation.[7]

TAKING A MULTIDISCIPLINARY APPROACH TO EVALUATION

Because the practice of infection prevention is the responsibility of everyone in the organization, having staff from throughout the facility involved in the continuous evaluation process will provide a broad overview of risks and concerns associated with reducing infections in patients, staff, physicians, visitors, and others.

Experience shows that promoting collaboration between individuals and departments results in developing broad-based solutions to problems and can result in both individual and corporate ownership. Multidisciplinary collaboration and a systems approach increase the likelihood of a successful IPC program.

Including others in the entire cycle, from risk assessment through evaluation, will develop teams that effectively move a specific issue from the risk column to successful and sustained resolution. The infection prevention and control staff should reinforce the importance of casting a wide net within the organization to identify and determine the seriousness of infection risks, assist with the prioritization process, develop appropriate goals and measurable objectives, and identify key partners in this process.

SUMMARY

The intent of the evaluation standard is to analyze the activities of an IPC program to determine what works well and what needs to be changed. A well-designed evaluation will also provide information to leadership on the program's challenges and successes.

Table 10-1. Infection Prevention and Control Committee Report

ANNUAL REPORT: EVALUATING SUCCESS IN MEETING OBJECTIVES OF THE PROGRAM

Risk	Objective	Strategies	Evaluation
Central line–associated bloodstream infections (CLABSIs) in intensive care unit (ICU) patients	Achieve zero CLABSIs for at least three months in the two ICUs	• Continue to promote CLABSI prevention bundle • Provide data on CLABSIs to ICU personnel weekly • Discuss results at weekly ICU performance improvement meeting	• Medical ICU attained zero CLABSIs during four months • Surgical ICU attained zero CLABSIs for two months • Target met in medical ICU (MICU) and almost met in surgical ICU • Continue to target zero and use this objective next year.
Pneumonia in ventilated patients in the MICU	Decrease the rate of ventilator-associated pneumonia (VAP) to at least the 25th percentile of NHSN	Staff educated in prevention procedures during June 2008: • Keep head of the bed at 30° angle • Use equipment according to Centers for Disease Control and Prevention (CDC) guidelines	• 2008 rate = 6.8 VAP/1,000 ventilator days • NHSN 25th percentile = 2.1 VAP/1,000 ventilator days • **Target not met** To decrease VAP rates, this objective will continue to be a focus for improvement in 2009.
Surgical site infections (SSIs) post–open reduction internal fixation (ORIF)	Decrease the rate of SSIs post-ORIF to < 2%	• CHG used to prepare surgical site as of January 2007 • Patients began taking a preprocedure shower with CHG as of March 2006 • # SSIs detected and rates provided to surgeons monthly	• Rate for 2008 = 1.1% • Rate for 2007 = 2.6% • Target met Objective will not be used next year, but surveillance will continue to monitor SSIs related to ORIF and take action if the rate increases to 2% or above.
Ventriculitis in patients with ventriculostomy	Decrease the rate of ventriculitis by at least 20%	• Strict insertion standards developed • Staff educated in April 2007	• Rate for 2008 = 3.5 infections/1,000 catheter days • Rate for 2007 = 4.6 infections/1,000 catheter days • Rate decrease from 2007 to 2008 = 23% • Target met Objective will not be used next year, but surveillance will continue to monitor ventriculitis and action will be taken if rate reaches 3.5 or more infections/1,000 catheter days.

(continued)

Table 10-1. Infection Prevention and Control Committee Report (continued)

Risk	Objective	Strategies	Evaluation
Nosocomial tuberculosis (TB) infection in staff and patients	Ensure no transmission of TB from patients to staff or other patients	• Policy revision, education, and nursing authority to isolate patients suspected of having TB promptly • TB test for all new staff to determine baseline and rule out existing TB	• 100% of new staff tested for TB infection • No cases of TB infection or disease occurred in a staff member or patient this past year • **Target met** Objective will not be used next year, but surveillance to monitor TB infections in patients and personnel is ongoing.
Hand hygiene compliance (HH)	Ensure HH compliance rate exceeds 85% on at least 90% clinical units	• Alcohol hand rub made available in September 2004 • Additional education provided • Administrator of patient care services served as champion for HH initiative • Compliance data sent to clinical units quarterly; instituted peer feedback • Provided reports on HH compliance to clinical units quarterly • Measured HH product use in addition to observations	• HH compliance rates met or exceeded 85% on 92% of units. • **Target met** A similar objective will be used next year to further increase the HH rate.
Influenza (flu) immunization in staff	Increase employee flu vaccination rates to achieve at least 70% of all eligible staff	• Flu vaccine offered to staff in the fall • Flu "clinics" held daily during the last week of October • Marketing campaign held	• Rate for 2008: 75% of staff received vaccine • **Target met** A similar objective will be used next year to further improve the flu vaccination rate.

This table shows how one organization reported the evaluation of its infection prevention and control (IPC) program objectives.

Source: Candace Friedman, M.P.H., C.I.C.; and Susan Slavish, B.S.N., M.P.H., C.I.C.

FURTHER RESOURCES

Refer to the following resources for helpful information on how to evaluate the effectiveness of an infection control program.

CD Tool

Tool 10-1: Johnson City Medical Center IPC Program Evaluation

Additional Readings

■ Centers for Disease Control and Prevention: Framework for program evaluation in public health. *MMWR Recomm Rep* 48(RR-11), 1999. http://www.cdc.gov/eval/framework.htm (accessed Feb. 18, 2009).

■ Friedman C., et al.: APIC/CHICA–Canada infection control and epidemiology: Professional and practice standards. *Am J Infect Control* 36:385–389, 2008.

■ Scheckler W.E., et al.: Requirements for infrastructure and essential activities of infection control and epidemiology in hospitals: A consensus panel report. *Am J Infect Control* 26:47–60, 1998.

REFERENCES

1. Bower J., Segarra-Newnham M., Tice A.: Selecting change implementation strategies. In Mayhall C.G. (ed.): *Hospital Epidemiology and Infection Control*, 3rd ed. Philadelphia: Lippincott-Williams & Wilkins, 2004, pp. 162–163.

2. De Feo J.A., Barnard W.: *JURAN Institute's Six Sigma Breakthrough and Beyond—Quality Performance Breakthrough Methods.* New York: McGraw-Hill Publishing Company Limited, 2005.

3. Womack J.P., Jones D.T., Roos D.: *The Machine That Changed the World: The Story of Lean Production.* New York: HarperBusiness, 1991.

4. Deming W.E.: *Out of the Crisis.* Cambridge, MA: MIT Center for Advanced Engineering Study, 1986.

5. Balachandran M.E.: *Effective Written Presentation.* Spring 2005. http://frank.mtsu.edu/~mbalacha/longreport.htm (accessed Oct. 11, 2009).

6. Stone P.W., et al.: The economic impact of infection control: Making the business case for increased infection control resources. *Am J Infect Control* 33:542–547, 2005.

7. Dunagan W.C., et al.: Making the business case for infection control: Pitfalls and opportunities. *Am J Infect Control* 30:86–92, 2002.

Chapter 11

Patient Safety and Performance Improvement

Kathleen Meehan Arias, M.S., C.I.C.

As discussed in Chapter 2, health care–associated infections (HAIs) are among the most common adverse events in health care and have long been recognized as being problematic for patient safety.[1,2] Because HAIs cause significant morbidity and mortality, infection prevention and control (IPC) must be an essential component of an organization's patient safety and performance improvement programs.

In 2004, The Joint Commission introduced National Patient Safety Goal (NPSG) 7 "reduce the risk of health care-associated infections," which focused on reducing the risk of HAIs through hand hygiene compliance and required organizations to manage identified cases of death or major loss of function related to an HAI as a sentinel event. In 2009, the Joint Commission made the following revisions to NPSG 7:

- Deleted sentinel events related to HAIs from the NPSG but retained the requirement to manage as sentinel events all identified cases of unanticipated death or major permanent loss of function related to an HAI under the sentinel event policy requirement in the "Improving Organization Performance" (PI) chapter
- Added three new requirements related to the following topics: multidrug-resistant organisms (MDROs), central line–associated bloodstream infections (CLABSIs), and surgical site infections (SSIs)

This chapter discusses strategies and interventions that health care organizations can use to support compliance with National Patient Safety Goal 7 and other National Patient Safety Goals that relate to infection prevention and control.

NATIONAL PATIENT SAFETY GOAL 7
Reduce the risk of health care–associated infections.

THE JOINT COMMISSION'S INFECTION PREVENTION NATIONAL PATIENT SAFETY GOAL

The purpose of the NPSG is to promote specific improvements in patient safety. In the case of NPSG 7, these improvements relate to preventing the spread of infections and responding to incidents that involve infections.

Because surveyors evaluate an organization's actual performance in meeting the NPSG requirements, not just the intent to meet them, organizations must not only implement strategies to prevent infection but must also develop a mechanism to ensure ongoing compliance with the strategies. As discussed in Chapter 10, an organization must then measure the effectiveness of its IPC program as a routine part of its performance improvement activities.

Because the risk of adverse health care events—including those that involve infections—is related to the types of care, treatment, and services provided by an organization, the NPSG and requirements are program specific. Therefore, organizations that are accredited by the Joint Commission must be aware of which requirements pertain to their setting. The health care programs to which NPSG 7 requirements apply are outlined in Table 11-1 on page 127.

TIP: *Because HAIs cause significant morbidity and mortality, infection prevention and control must be an essential component of an organization's patient safety and performance improvement programs.*

EXPLORING NATIONAL PATIENT SAFETY GOAL 7

As previously mentioned, NPSG 7 addresses four topics related to infection control and prevention:

1. Hand hygiene
2. Preventing HAIs related to MDROs
3. Preventing CLABSIs
4. Preventing SSIs

The following sections examine these topics and their associated requirements more closely.

TIP: *It is not possible to prevent all HAIs. However, health care organizations that have aggressively targeted reducing the occurrence of specific HAIs for which there are known infection prevention interventions, such as CLABSIs, have demonstrated infection rates close to zero—a target that has long been considered unattainable.[3]*

Hand Hygiene Compliance

> **NPSG.07.01.01:**
>
> Comply with current World Health Organization (WHO) or Centers for Disease Control and Prevention (CDC) hand hygiene guidelines.
>
> EP 1: The [organization] complies with current World Health Organization (WHO) or Centers for Disease Control and Prevention (CDC) hand hygiene guidelines. Note: [Organizations] are required to comply with 1A, 1B, and 1C of the WHO or CDC guidelines.

Although proper hand hygiene has been shown to reduce the risk of infection, many studies show that hand hygiene compliance by health care personnel is poor. By implementing the Centers for Disease Control and Prevention (CDC)[4] or World Health Organization (WHO)[5] hand hygiene guidelines, health care organizations will reduce the risk of transmission of infectious agents and the occurrence of HAIs.

Organizations that have successfully improved hand hygiene compliance have used a multimodal, multidisciplinary approach that includes strategies such as the following:

- Educating personnel, patients, residents, and visitors about the importance of hand hygiene and how to properly clean hands
- Providing appropriate hand hygiene facilities and products in convenient locations
- Hanging posters and other reminders to clean hands by sinks, in restrooms, and in other strategic locations
- Encouraging care recipients and families to speak up and ask health care personnel to clean their hands
- Creating and implementing rewards programs
- Measuring compliance with hand hygiene procedures and providing feedback to health care personnel on their performance
- Ensuring management and leadership support of hand hygiene programs
- Using medical staff role models
- Instituting a culture of patient safety and leadership and health care worker accountability[6-8]

To fully demonstrate compliance with NPSG.07.01.01, organizations must have evidence that they have selected either the CDC or WHO guidelines and must have identified, implemented, and monitored compliance with policies and practices based on the CDC or WHO guidelines (Category 1A, 1B, and 1C recommendations). As part of this effort, organizations should set a goal to improve hand hygiene compliance, use performance measurement tools, and provide feedback of compliance rates to health care providers. (The "Further Resources" section at the end of this chapter contains information and links to resources that can be used to promote and measure compliance with the CDC and WHO hand hygiene guidelines.)

Preventing Health Care–Associated Infections Related to Multidrug-Resistant Organisms

> **NPSG.07.03.01:**
>
> Implement evidence-based practices to prevent health care–associated infections due to multidrug–resistant organisms in the [organization].
>
> *Note 1:* This requirement applies to, but is not limited to, epidemiologically significant organisms such as methicillin-resistant *Staphylococcus aureus* (MRSA), *Clostridium difficile* (CDI), vancomycin-resistant Enterococcus (VRE), and multiple-drug-resistant gram-negative bacteria.

Table 11-1. Programs to Which National Patient Safety Goal 7 Requirement Apply

NPSG Requirement	Program							
	Amb Care	Behavioral Health	Critical Access Hospital	Home Care	Hospital	Lab	LTC	Office-Based Surg
07.01.01 Hand hygiene	✓	✓	✓	✓	✓	✓	✓	✓
07.03.01 MDRO			✓		✓			
07.04.01 CLABSI			✓		✓		✓*	
07.05.01 SSI	✓		✓		✓			✓

Legend: Amb care, ambulatory care; Lab, laboratory; LTC, long term care; Office based surg, office-based surgery; MDROs, multidrug-resistant organisms; CLABSIs, central line–associated bloodstream infections; SSIs, surgical site infections.

* Effective July 1, 2010, for Medicaid/Medicare Certification–based long term care.

Note 2: Surveillance may be targeted, and not organizationwide.

EP 5: Conduct periodic risk assessments for multidrug-resistant organisms' acquisition and transmission. (See also IC.01.03.01, EPs 1–5.)

EP 6: Based on the results of the risk assessment, educate staff and licensed independent practitioners about health care–associated infections, multidrug-resistant organisms, and prevention strategies at hire and annually thereafter.

Note: The education provided recognizes the diverse roles of staff and licensed independent practitioners and is consistent with their roles within the organization. (*See also* HR.01.05.03, EP 4.)

EP 7: Educate patients, and their families as needed, who are infected or colonized with a multidrug-resistant organism about health care–associated infection strategies.

EP 8: Implement a surveillance program for multidrug-resistant organisms based on the risk assessment.

EP 9: Measure and monitor multidrug-resistant organism prevention processes and outcomes including the following:
- Multidrug-resistant organism infection rates using evidence-based metrics
- Compliance with evidence-based guidelines or best practices
- Evaluation of the education program provided to staff and licensed independent practitioners

EP 10: Provide multidrug-resistant organism surveillance data to key stakeholders, including leaders, licensed independent practitioners, nursing staff, and other clinicians.

EP 11: Implement policies and practices aimed at reducing the risk of transmitting multidrug-resistant organisms that meet regulatory requirements and are aligned with evidence-based standards (for example, the Centers for Disease Control and Prevention [CDC] and/or professional organization guidelines).

EP 12: When indicated by the risk assessment, implement a laboratory-based alert system that identifies new patients with multidrug-resistant organisms. The alert system may be either manual or electronic or a combination of both of these methods. *Note:* The alert system may use telephones, faxes, pagers, automated and secure electronic alerts, or a combination of these methods.

EP 13: When indicated by the risk assessment, implement an alert system that identifies readmitted or transferred multidrug-resistant organism–positive patients. *Note:* The alert system information may exist in a separate electronic database or may be integrated into the admission system. The alert system may be either manual or electronic or both.

The presence of MDROs that can cause infections is on the rise in health care organizations, specifically within acute care settings. The following strategies can be used to prevent infections due to MDROs and to support compliance with NPSG.07.03.01, EPs 5 through 13:

- *Conduct a risk assessment.* To help identify the presence of MDROs, an organization should periodically assess the occurrence of MDROs in patients, personnel, and the community and should document findings. Organizations should identify which MDROs and other organisms are considered "epidemiologically significant" in patients and personnel, should incorporate surveillance findings related to epidemiologically significant organisms into risk assessments, and should document these findings in the infection prevention and control plan (as discussed in Chapter 4). An MDRO risk assessment can be integrated into the overall IPC program risk assessment or can be a stand-alone document.
- *Educate personnel.* To ensure that staff understand how to prevent the spread of MDROs, organizations should develop and implement education activities about HAIs, MDROs, and infection prevention strategies. These education activities should be based on the risk assessments and surveillance findings discussed previously and should be provided to personnel, including licensed independent practitioners, at the time of hire and annually thereafter. An organization may want to consider incorporating information on MDRO infection, transmission, and prevention into its new employee orientation and an intranet learning course that nurses and other staff are required to complete annually. Education and training should be

based on staff members' education levels and role in the organization.

Once training is under way, organizations should evaluate the effectiveness of the training by monitoring compliance with protocols and the occurrence of colonization and infection with MDROs. For example, organizations should consider measuring compliance with contact precautions used to prevent transmission of MDROs and to provide compliance rates to the groups of personnel observed.

- *Educate patients.* Organizations must provide education about HAIs, MDROs, and infection prevention strategies to patients infected or colonized with an MDRO, and to their family members as needed. Vehicles for this education include a pamphlet, video, scripted discussion, or a combination of these, depending on the status of the patient and the learning levels of the patient and family or advocate. (Refer to the "Further Resources" section at the end of this chapter for sample patient education materials.)
- *Conduct surveillance.* Organizations should ensure that their infection surveillance programs have identified those organisms considered epidemiologically significant and should monitor laboratory reports for their occurrence. For example, based on organization and community surveillance data from previous years, an organization may want to monitor the occurrence of methicillin-resistant *Staphylococcus aureus* (MRSA), vancomycin-resistant *enterococcus* (VRE), *Clostridium difficile*, and gram-negative bacilli that produce extended spectrum beta lactamase (ESBLs) in patients.
- *Measure and monitor.* To help with measuring and monitoring, organizations should use recognized surveillance methodology and criteria, such as those of the National Healthcare Safety Network (NHSN), to identify patients infected and colonized with epidemiologically significant organisms.[9] In addition, organizations should conduct surveillance for MDROs in accordance with evidence-based recommendations and guidelines, such as those of the NHSN, the CDC Healthcare Infection Control Practices Advisory Committee (HICPAC), and the Society for Healthcare Epidemiology of America (SHEA).[9–13] For example, organizations should use the methodology in the NHSN's *MDRO and* Clostridium difficile-*Associated Disease (CDAD) Module* to measure both infection

rates for MRSA and compliance with active surveillance testing for MRSA.[11] Likewise, organizations may want to consider maintaining an electronic line list of patients with newly recovered MDRO isolates by entering data on these patients into an electronic spreadsheet.[13] Because some states require specific surveillance activities and reports for specific organisms, an organization should ensure that its surveillance program complies with these and other applicable requirements.

Once surveillance findings are available, organizations should use these findings to evaluate the effectiveness of staff education programs. For instance, if several patients on one patient care unit develop infection and colonization with VRE and observations of the staff reveal lack of compliance with contact precautions, staff should be reeducated on appropriate practices used for contact precautions and laboratory reports should continue to be reviewed for the occurrence of new cases.

TIP: *Organizations should monitor both outcomes (such as MDRO infection and colonization rates) and processes (such as compliance with hand hygiene practices and contact precautions used for patients with an MDRO). See the "Further Resources" section for ideas on how to do this.*

■ *Provide surveillance data to stakeholders.* Organizations should provide MDRO surveillance data and findings to personnel involved in infection prevention activities, especially key stakeholders such as clinical leaders, licensed independent practitioners, nursing staff, and other clinicians. Information should be shared on what these individuals can do to prevent HAIs and the transmission of MDROs. For example, an infection preventionist can present surveillance findings and infection prevention recommendations to the patient safety and performance improvement committee at least once a year. In addition, infection preventionists should work with quality and safety personnel to ensure that accurate HAI data are routinely shared with executive leaders and governance, because the leaders of the health care organization may need to provide additional support and/or assist with removing barriers that impact patient risk for developing an HAI.

Furthermore, by sharing these data with leaders, leaders can appropriately reward and recognize staff performance that contributed to lowering the incidence of HAIs.

■ *Create policies and practices.* Organizations should develop and implement infection prevention policies and procedures that meet applicable regulatory requirements and are aligned with evidence-based standards, professional organization guidelines, and best practices.[12,14,15] (Refer to the "Further Resources" section for guidance.)

■ *Implement an alert system.* When indicated by the risk assessment, organizations should implement a system that identifies readmitted or transferred patients that have an MDRO and that notifies the infection preventionist and direct care providers.[12,14,15] This alert system can be manual, electronic, or communicated by phone, e-mail, or other methods.

Preventing Central Line–Associated Bloodstream Infections

NPSG.07.04.01:
Implement best practices or evidence-based guidelines to prevent central line–associated bloodstream infections.

Note 1: This requirement covers short- and long-term central venous catheters and peripherally inserted central catheter (PICC) lines.

EP 5: Educate health care workers who are involved in these procedures about health care–associated infections, central line–associated bloodstream infections, and the importance of prevention. Education occurs upon hire, annually thereafter, and when involvement in these procedures is added to an individual's job responsibilities.

EP 6: Prior to insertion of a central venous catheter, educate patients and, as needed, their families about central line–associated bloodstream infection prevention.

EP 7: Implement policies and practices aimed at reducing the risk of central line–associated bloodstream infections that meet regulatory requirements and are aligned with evidence-based standards (for example, the Centers for Disease Control and Prevention [CDC] and/or professional organization guidelines).

EP 8: Conduct periodic risk assessments for surgical site infections, measure central line–associated bloodstream infection rates, monitor compliance with best practices or evidence-based guidelines, and evaluate the effectiveness of prevention efforts.

EP 9: Provide central line–associated bloodstream infection rate data and prevention outcome measures to key stakeholders including leaders, licensed independent practitioners, nursing staff, and other clinicians.

EP 10: Use a catheter checklist and a standardized protocol for central venous catheter insertion.

EP 11: Perform hand hygiene prior to catheter insertion or manipulation.

EP 12: For adult patients, do not insert catheters into the femoral vein unless other sites are unavailable.

EP 13: Use a standardized supply cart or kit that is all inclusive for the insertion of central venous catheters.

EP 14: Use a standardized protocol for maximum sterile barrier precautions during central venous catheter insertion.

EP 15: Use a chlorhexidine-based antiseptic for skin preparation during central venous catheter insertion in patients over two months of age, unless contraindicated.

EP 16: Use a standardized protocol to disinfect catheter hubs and injection ports before accessing the ports.

EP 17: Evaluate all central venous catheters routinely and remove nonessential catheters.

Each year, nearly 250,000 CLABSIs occur in U.S. hospitals,[14] and many of these are associated with central vascular catheters (CVCs). Such infections can lead to increased hospital stays and sometimes mortality. The following strategies can be used to prevent CLABSIs and to support compliance with NPSG.07.04.01, EPs 5 through 17:

- *Educate personnel.* Organizations should develop and implement education activities about CLABSIs, the importance of preventing CLABSIs, and infection prevention strategies. These education activities should be based on periodic risk assessments and surveillance findings, and organizations should provide these activities to the personnel involved in CVC insertion and care, including licensed independent practitioners. Such activities should be provided at the time of hire and annually thereafter and when CVC insertion or care activities are added to an individual's job responsibilities. For example, a community teaching hospital can include information on CLABSI rates and central line insertion protocols in its new resident orientation program and can require all personnel involved in central line insertion to demonstrate competency annually, according to their job responsibilities.

- *Educate patients.* Prior to insertion of a CVC, staff should provide education to patients (and their families as needed). Such education could be in the form of a brochure, video, or scripted discussion, depending on the circumstances and needs of the patient and family. (The "Further Resources" section provides a variety of resources for patient education materials.)

- *Create policies and practices.* As with other types of infection prevention and control policies, CLABSI policies and practices should meet applicable regulatory requirements and should be aligned with evidence-based standards, professional organization guidelines, and best practices.[15,16] Examples of best practices include the following:
  — Using maximal sterile barriers during insertion
  — Creating and implementing a checklist to assure all required steps are completed per policy
  — Maintaining a cart or kit that contains all the necessary supplies for the procedure (*See* the "Further Resources" section for more information.)

- *Conduct risk assessments, surveillance, and evaluations.* An organization's infection surveillance program should monitor the occurrence of CLABSIs in its patient population based on the results of periodic risk assessments. This monitoring effort should use recognized surveillance methodology and criteria, such as that of the NHSN, to identify patients with CLABSIs.[10] The surveillance program must include monitoring of all central lines, not just those in patients in the intensive care unit (ICU). (*Note*: Organizations must ensure that the surveillance program meets state and other agency data collection and reporting requirements as discussed in Chapter 7.)

Organizations should incorporate surveillance findings related to CLABSIs into the periodic and annual risk assessments and the infection prevention and control plan as discussed in Chapter 4.

Organizations should also evaluate the effectiveness of CLABSI prevention activities and education efforts by monitoring the occurrence of CLABSIs and compliance with CLABSI infection prevention practices, such as hand hygiene and use of maximal barrier precautions for CVC insertion. Evaluation findings should be reported in the annual assessment of the IPC program.

■ *Provide surveillance data.* As with data on MDROs, organizations should provide CLABSI rates and data on compliance with infection prevention protocols to appropriate personnel, such as staff members involved in CVC insertion and care and other key stakeholders (fir example, clinical leaders, licensed independent practitioners, nursing staff). For example, organizations may want to present CLABSI rates and data on compliance with insertion protocols to the personnel in those units that care for patients with a CVC and to managers and medical staff at the units' quality improvement committee meetings. As noted previously, it is important to ensure that the data are also shared with the leaders of the organization.

■ *Ensure that standardized CVC insertion and care protocols are implemented.* Such protocols should include the following:
— A CVC insertion checklist (*See* the "Further Resources" section for examples of CVC insertion checklists.)
— Hand hygiene prior to insertion and manipulation
— Optimal catheter site selection that includes restriction of femoral vein use unless other sites are not available
— A standardized cart or kit that contains all of the supplies needed for CVC insertion

— Maximal sterile barrier precautions (use of sterile gloves, sterile gown, large sterile drape, mask/face shield, and cap)
— Chlorhexidine-based antiseptic for skin prep (in patients over two months old) unless contraindicated
— Disinfecting catheter hubs and injection ports

One way to ensure the use of standardized protocols is to create a CLABSI bundle for CVC insertion that includes all these elements.

■ *Remove nonessential CVCs.* Organizations should establish a mechanism for routinely evaluating all patients with CVCs and removing nonessential catheters. One method to ensure that this occurs is to incorporate daily evaluation for need into the nursing care plan or medical staff rounds for all patients with central lines and to include a follow-up mechanism to ensure prompt CVC removal when no longer needed.

Preventing Surgical Site Infections

NPSG.07.05.01

Implement best practices for preventing surgical site infections.

EP 5: Educate health care workers involved in surgical procedures about health care–associated infections, surgical site infections, and the importance of prevention. Education occurs upon hire, annually thereafter, and when involvement in surgical procedures is added to an individual's job responsibilities.

EP 6: Prior to all surgical procedures, educate patients and their families, as needed, who are undergoing a surgical procedure about surgical site infection prevention.

EP 7: Implement policies and practices aimed at reducing the risk of surgical site infections that meet regulatory requirements and are aligned with evidence-based standards (for example, the Centers for Disease Control and Prevention [CDC] and/or professional organization guidelines).

EP 8: Conduct periodic risk assessments for surgical site infections, select surgical site infection measures using best practices or evidence-based guidelines, monitor compliance with best practices or evidence-based guidelines, and evaluate the effectiveness of prevention efforts.

EP 9: Surgical site infection rates are measured for the first 30 days following procedures that do not involve inserting implantable devices and for the first year following procedures involving implantable devices.

EP 10: Provide surgical site infection rate data and prevention outcome measures to key stakeholders, including leaders, licensed independent practitioners, nursing staff, and other clinicians.

EP 11: Administer antimicrobial agents for prophylaxis used for a particular procedure or disease according to evidence-based standards and guidelines for best practices.

EP 12: When hair removal is necessary, use clippers or depilatories. *Note:* Shaving is an inappropriate hair removal method.

As with other types of infections, the prevalence of SSIs in health care organizations is higher than it should be. In addition, the consequences of these infections can be devastating to patients, staff members, and organizations' bottom lines. The following strategies can be used to prevent SSIs and support compliance with NPSG.07.05.01, EPs 5 through 12:

- *Educate personnel.* As with other types of infections, organizations should develop and implement education activities about SSIs, the importance of preventing SSIs, and infection prevention strategies. These activities should be based on periodic risk assessments and surveillance findings and should be provided to personnel involved in surgical procedures upon hire, annually, and when involvement in surgical procedures is added to an individual's job responsibilities. For example, organizations may want to implement an orientation program on SSI prevention that includes both new employees hired for the perioperative area and those personnel who are transferred to the perioperative unit from another area of the organization.
- *Educate patients.* Patients (and their families, as needed) should receive education prior to all surgical

procedures. This education can take a variety of forms. For example, in addition to patient education brochures, an organization can develop Internet-based education videos on what to expect before, during, and after surgery and how to recognize and prevent infection. (*See* the "Further Resources" section for samples of patient education materials.)

- *Create and implement policies and practices.* As with other types of infections, organizations should develop and implement SSI prevention policies and procedures that meet applicable regulatory requirements and that are aligned with evidence-based standards, professional organization guidelines, and best practices.[17–19] For example, organizations should implement antibiotic prophylaxis protocols aligned with those in the Surgical Care Improvement Project (SCIP). (*See* the "Further Resources" section for guidance on creating policies and practices.)
- *Conduct risk assessments, surveillance, and evaluations.* Organizations should ensure that their infection surveillance programs are based on periodic assessments of their patient populations and the types of surgical procedures performed. As with other types of infections, organizations should monitor both outcomes (number of SSIs) and processes related to SSI prevention (for example, adherence to appropriate antimicrobial prophylaxis). Organizations should ensure that their surveillance programs use recognized surveillance methodology and criteria, such as that of the NHSN, to identify patients with SSIs.[10] The surveillance program should also meet state, Centers for Medicare & Medicaid Services (CMS), and other data collection and reporting requirements, as discussed in Chapter 7.

As with other infections, findings related to SSIs should be included in the organization's periodic and annual risk assessments and the infection prevention and control plan. Organizations should evaluate the effectiveness of SSI prevention activities and education efforts and report evaluation findings in the annual assessment of the IPC program.

- *Provide surveillance data to stakeholders.* Organizations should provide SSI rates and data on compliance with infection prevention protocols to key stakeholders, such as clinical leaders, licensed independent practitioners, nursing staff, and other clinicians, including information on what they can do to prevent

SSIs. For example, the infection preventionist can report procedure-specific SSI rates and data on compliance with the SCIP measures to the perioperative care committee on a regular basis and include recommendations for improving compliance with antibiotic prophylaxis as needed.

MANAGING SENTINEL EVENTS RELATED TO HEALTH CARE–ASSOCIATED INFECTIONS

As mentioned in Chapter 1, approximately 1.7 million HAIs occurred in U.S. hospitals in 2002, and an estimated 99,000 deaths were determined to be caused by or associated with these infections.[20] HAIs that may be attributable causes of unanticipated death or major permanent loss of function should be identified during routine surveillance activities, and these cases should be individually evaluated. If an unexpected death or major loss of function is determined to be due to an HAI, the case should be managed as a sentinel event.

Although sentinel events related to an HAI have been deleted from the NPSGs, the Joint Commission still requires organizations to manage as sentinel events all identified cases of unanticipated death or major permanent loss of function related to an HAI. Each Joint Commission accreditation manual contains standards in the "Improving Organization Performance" (PI) chapter that relate to the management of sentinel events. These standards are PI.1.10, PI.2.20, PI.2.30, and PI.3.10.

The sentinel event policy and procedure states that accredited organizations are expected to identify sentinel events "occurring in the organization or associated with services that the organization provides, or provides for. Appropriate response includes conducting a timely, thorough, and credible root cause analysis; developing an action plan designed to implement improvements to reduce risk; implementing the improvements; and monitoring the effectiveness of those improvements."[21]

The following strategies can be used to support compliance with the Joint Commission's sentinel event requirements:

- *Identify and analyze potential HAI-related sentinel events.* Organizations must ensure that their routine surveillance system is capable of identifying patients or residents who may have died unexpectedly or suffered major permanent loss of function as a consequence of an HAI. In addition, organizations should ensure that these cases are referred to the risk manager, patient safety coordinator, or other person who coordinates review of adverse events, including sentinel events.

Organizations should develop a process for analyzing cases identified as potential HAI-related sentinel events and should incorporate criteria to differentiate between those patients or residents who die *with* an HAI and those who die *due to* an HAI. For example, a sentinel event is likely to have occurred when an otherwise healthy patient admitted for an elective operative procedure develops an SSI, becomes septic, and dies. However, if an immunocompromised or elderly person with multiple comorbidities develops an HAI and dies, the death may be related to the underlying diseases and/or the HAI, and the occurrence of a sentinel event is more difficult to determine.

Organizations can use a variety of resources to help with analyzing sentinel events due to HAIs. For example, Carrico and Ramirez have published a comprehensive resource, that includes algorithms, forms, and sample fishbone diagrams.[22] Likewise, a link to a document produced by the Association for Professionals in Infection Control and Epidemiology (APIC) that includes infection-related sentinel event analysis questions and sample scenarios can be found in the "Further Resources" section at the end of this chapter.

- *If a sentinel event is identified, conduct a thorough and credible root cause analysis (RCA).* An RCA is a performance improvement tool that is used to methodically study an adverse event to identify possible causal factors and root causes that could have contributed to the occurrence of an event. The purpose of doing an RCA is to identify improvements in systems or processes of care that can be implemented to prevent a similar event from occurring. Because there are many different techniques and tools for performing an RCA, organizations should determine how they will define a *sentinel event* and should establish mechanisms to identify, report, analyze, and manage these events. Organizations should consider using a multidisciplinary team to conduct sentinel event analyses and RCAs and using a stepwise approach. To help with this process, the Joint

Commission has forms and tools for conducting an RCA and developing an action plan at http://www.jointcommission.org/SentinelEvents/Forms.

- *Develop an action plan.* Once an RCA has been completed—systems and practices involved have been reviewed and analyzed and contributing risk factors and root causes have been identified—the organization should develop and implement strategies aimed at preventing a similar event from occurring. The organization should develop an action plan based on a literature review of similar events, recognized infection prevention practices, and appropriate standards. It should include in the action plan measures of effectiveness for the strategies to be implemented. A framework for an action plan has been developed by the Joint Commission (http://www.jointcommission.org/SentinelEvents/Forms) and built upon by APIC (*see* Tool 11-1 in the "CD Tools" section.)

- *Implement strategies for improvement.* Once an action plan has been developed, organizations should implement the strategies outlined in the action plan to reduce risk in all areas where applicable, not just where the event occurred. For example, if a previously healthy patient admitted to the ICU contracts MRSA infection at a CVC line site, develops sepsis, and dies, this would be considered a sentinel event. Consequently, the risk reduction/performance improvement interventions identified should be implemented in all of the areas that care for patients with CVCs and not just in the ICU.

- *Monitor and determine the effectiveness of the strategies.* Once strategies have been implemented, an organization must monitor the effectiveness of those strategies. For example, after implementing actions to reduce infections among patients with CVCs, an organization should conduct surveillance to identify cases of CVC line site infection. If any are found, the organization should reinforce infection prevention practices for CVC line insertion and site care.

SUMMARY

Infection prevention and control is an integral component of an organization's patient safety and performance improvement programs. The interventions discussed in this chapter focus on the implementation of evidence-based practices that have been shown to reduce the risk of infection, thus improving patient safety.

Infection preventionists play an essential role in improving performance and supporting a culture of patient safety. As discussed in the previous chapters of this workbook, by collaborating with others in the organization to rigorously and accurately measure outcomes and processes of care, provide performance measurement findings to those who can improve the quality of care, and promote the use of feasible and effective infection prevention interventions, an infection preventionist can advance the changes needed to improve health care quality.

FURTHER RESOURCES

The following sections provide further information on infection control and patient safety and can serve as a valuable reference in assisting your organization with infection prevention and NPSG compliance efforts.

CD Tools

Tool 11-1: APIC: Integrating Sentinel Event Analysis into Your Infection Control Practice, 2004. Available at http://www.apic.org/AM/Template.cfm?Section=Search&section=Position_Statements1&template=/CM/ContentDisplay.cfm&ContentFileID=6148.

Tool 11-2: Implementation Work Plan for NPSG 07.04.01—CLABSIs—Driscoll Children's Hospital

Tool 11-3: Implementation Work Plan for NPSG 07.05.01—SSIs—Driscoll Children's Hospital

Tool 11-4: Hand Hygiene Education and Monitoring Program—Novant Health

Tool 11-5: Dietary Department—2009 Hand Hygiene Monitoring Tool: Peer Audit—Wilson Memorial Hospital

Tool 11-6: 2009 Surgery Department Hand Hygiene Monitoring Tool: Peer Audit—Wilson Memorial Hospital

Tool 11-7: Central Line Procedural Checklist—Bloomington Hospital of Orange County

Tool 11-8: Central Line Insertion and Daily Monitoring Form—Placentia Linda Hospital

Tool 11-9: National Healthcare Safety Network *Central Line Insertion Practices Adherence Monitoring* form. Available in the NHSN Document Library at http://www.cdc.gov/nhsn/dataCollectForms.html.

Tool 11-10: Preventing Surgical Site Infections—Cooley Dickinson Hospital

Tool 11-11: CLABSI Prevention Bundle. California Children's Services and California Children's Hospital Association Neonatal Intensive Care Unit Collaborative for the Prevention of CLABSI. Project information at http://www.dhcs.ca.gov/ProvGovPart/initiatives/nqi/Pages/default.aspx.

Additional Readings
Hand Hygiene
- Centers for Disease Control and Prevention: *Hand Hygiene in Healthcare Setting*. http://www.cdc.gov/handhygiene/index.html.
- Community and Hospital Infection Control Association–Canada (CHICA–Canada); *Links and Resources: Information About Hand Hygiene*. http://www.chica.org/links_handhygiene.html.
- Hand Hygiene Resource Center: *Tools*. http://www.handhygiene.org/educational_tools.asp. Provides hand hygiene monitoring tools.
- Institute for Healthcare Improvement: *How-to Guide: Improving Hand Hygiene*. http://www.ihi.org/IHI/Topics/HealthcareAssociatedInfections/InfectionsGeneral/Tools/HowtoGuideImprovingHandHygiene.htm. Includes protocol and forms for measuring compliance.
- The Joint Commission: *Hand Hygiene: Toolkit for Implementing the National Patient Safety Goal*. Oakbrook Terrace, IL: Joint Commission Resources, 2008.
- The Joint Commission: *Measuring Hand Hygiene Adherence: Overcoming the Challenges*. 2009. http://www.jointcommission.org/NR/rdonlyres/68B9CB2F-789F-49DB-9E3F-2FB387666BCC/0/hh_monograph.pdf.
- University of Geneva Hospitals: *Hospisafe Home Page*. http://www.hopisafe.ch.

- The National Center for Patient Safety (NCPS), Department of Veterans Affairs (VA) Veterans Health Administration (VHA): *VHA Hand Hygiene Tools*. http://www.va.gov/NCPS/SafetyTopics/HandHygiene/index.html#tools.
- World Health Organization: *Global Patient Safety Challenge*. http://www.who.int/patientsafety/challenge/en/.
- World Health Organization: *WHO Guidelines on Hand Hygiene in Health Care*, 2009. http://whqlibdoc.who.int/publications/2009/9789241597906_eng.pdf.

Sentinel Events
- The Joint Commission: *Sentinel Events*. http://www.jointcommission.org/SentinelEvents/. Information, policies, procedures, forms and tools for recognizing, investigating, and responding to a sentinel event.
- Joint Commission on Accreditation of Healthcare Organizations: *Root Cause Analysis in Health Care: Tools and Techniques*, 3rd ed. Oakbrook Terrace, IL: Joint Commission Resources, 2005.

Multidrug-Resistant Organisms
- Association for Professionals in Infection Control and Epidemiology (APIC): *Guide to the Elimination of Clostridium difficile in Healthcare Settings*. Washington, DC: APIC, 2008. Available at http://www.apic.org/EliminationGuides.
- Association for Professionals in Infection Control and Epidemiology (APIC): *Guide to the Elimination of Methicillin-Resistant* Staphylococcus aureus *(MRSA) Transmission in Hospital Settings*. Washington, DC: APIC, 2007. Available at http://www.apic.org/EliminationGuides.
- Association for Professionals in Infection Control and Epidemiology (APIC): *Guide to the Elimination of Methicillin-Resistant* Staphylococcus aureus *(MRSA) Transmission in Hospital Settings. California Supplement—2009*. Available at http://www.apic.org/EliminationGuides.
- Centers for Disease Control and Prevention: *NHSN MDRO and* C. difficile *surveillance module*. http://www.cdc.gov/nhsn/mdro_cdad.html.
- Centers for Disease Control and Prevention: *Get Smart: Know When Antibiotics Work*. http://www.cdc.gov/drugresistance/community/index.htm.

- Centers for Disease Control and Prevention: *Antibiotic/Antimicrobial Resistance.* http://www.cdc.gov/drugresistance/index.htm.
- Centers for Disease Control and Prevention: *National MRSA Education Initiative: Preventing MRSA Skin Infections.* www.cdc.gov/mrsa. Includes brochures, fact sheets, posters, Web graphics, and a treatment algorithm related to MRSA skin and soft tissue infections.
- Centers for Disease Control and Prevention: *Campaign to Prevent Antimicrobial Resistance in Healthcare Settings.* http://www.cdc.gov/drugresistance/healthcare. Includes information, tools, brochures, and slide sets.
- Centers for Disease Control and Prevention: *National Healthcare Safety Network (NHSN).* http://www.cdc.gov/nhsn/.

Central Line–Associated Bloodstream Infection Prevention

- Association for Professionals in Infection Control and Epidemiology (APIC): *Eliminating Catheter-Related Infections. A Guide for More Effective Infection Prevention and Control.* (Contains print-based User's Guide, DVD demonstrating CVC and PICC line insertion and care, tear-off pads with CVC insertion checklist and patient education fact sheet on avoiding infections at home with a CVC. This is a CME/CNE certified program.)
- Institute for Health Care Improvement: *Getting Started Kit: Prevent Central Line Infections; How-to Guide.* http://www.aap.org/visit/ IHI.CentralLinesHowtoGuideFINAL52505.pdf.
- The Joint Commission: *Clinical Care Improvement Strategies: Preventing Central Line Bloodstream Infections.* Oakbrook Terrace, IL: Joint Commission Resources, 2009.

Surgical Site Infection Prevention

- Centers for Medicare and Medicaid Services: *Surgical Care Improvement Project (SCIP).* http://www.qualitynet.org (search for SCIP).
- American College of Surgeons: *Patient Education: Partners in Surgical Care.* http://www.facs.org/patienteducation/index.html.

- Association for Professionals in Infection Control and Epidemiology (APIC): *Guide for the Prevention of Mediastinitis Surgical Site Infection Following Cardiac Surgery.* Washington, DC: APIC, 2008. Available at http://www.apic.org/EliminationGuides.
- Institute for Healthcare Improvement: *Getting Started Kit: Prevent Surgical Site Infections, How-to Guide.* 2008. http://www.ihi.org/NR/rdonlyres/ C54B5133-F4BB-4360-A3E4-2952C08C9B59/ 0/SSIHowtoGuide.doc.

Patient Safety and Performance Measurement and Improvement

- Agency for Healthcare Research and Quality: *Quality and Patient Safety.* http://www.ahrq.gov/qual.
- Centers for Medicare & Medicaid Services: *Quality of Care Center.* http://www.cms.hhs.gov/center/quality.asp.
- Institute for Healthcare Improvement: *Home page.* http://www.ihi.org/IHI/. Provides performance improvement references and tools.
- National Patient Safety Foundation (NPSF): *Home page.* http://www.npsf.org. Links to many patient safety resources and patient education materials though the NPSF Resource Center.
- National Quality Forum: *Home Page.* http://www.qualityforum.org. Provides quality and performance measures.

Patient Education Materials Not Noted Elsewhere in This Chapter

- Society for Healthcare Epidemiology of America: *Patient Guides on Health Care–Associated Infections.* http://www.shea-online.org/about/patientguides.cfm. Includes CLABSI, SSI, *C. difficile,* and MRSA.

REFERENCES

1. Burke J.P.: Infection control—A problem for patient safety. *N Engl J Med* 348:651–656, Feb. 13, 2003.
2. Leape L.L., et al.: The nature of adverse events in hospitalized patients. Results of the Harvard Medical Practice Study II. *N Engl J Med* 324:377–384, Feb. 7, 1991.
3. Pronovost P.: Interventions to decrease catheter-related bloodstream infections in the ICU: The Keystone Intensive Care Unit Project. *Am J Infect Control* 36, Dec. 2008. http://www.ajicjournal.org/article/S0196-6553(08)00793-1/ abstract (accessed Mar. 4, 2009).

4. Centers for Disease Control and Prevention: Guideline for hand hygiene in health-care settings. Recommendations of the Healthcare Infection Control Practices Advisory Committee and the HICPAC/SHEA/APIC/IDSA Hand Hygiene Task Force. *MMWR* Recomm Rep 51(RR16), Oct. 25, 2002. http://www.cdc.gov/mmwr/preview/mmwrhtml/rr5116a1.htm (accessed Feb. 21, 2009).

5. World Health Organization: *WHO Guidelines on Hand Hygiene in Health Care.* 2009. http://whqlibdoc.who.int/publications/2009/9789241597906_eng.pdf (accessed July 21, 2009).

6. Lankford M.G., et al.: Influence of role models and hospital design on the hand hygiene of health-care workers. *Emerg Infect Dis,* Feb. 2003. http://www.cdc.gov/ncidod/EID/vol9no2/02-0249.htm (accessed Feb. 21, 2009).

7. Pittet D.: Improving adherence to hand hygiene practice: A multidisciplinary approach. *Emerg Infect Dis,* Mar.–Apr. 2001. http://www.cdc.gov/ncidod/eid/vol7no2/pittet.htm (accessed Feb. 21, 2009).

8. The Joint Commission: *Speak Up: Five Things You Can Do to Prevent Infection.* http://www.jointcommission.org/PatientSafety/SpeakUp/speak_up_ic.htm (accessed Feb 21, 2009).

9. Centers for Disease Control and Prevention: *National Healthcare Safety Network (NHSN) Manual: Patient Safety Component Protocols.* http://www.cdc.gov/nhsn/library.html#psc (accessed Feb. 24, 2009).

10. Siegel J.D., et al.: *Multidrug-Resistant Organisms in Healthcare Settings,* 2006. Healthcare Infection Control Practices Advisory Committee. http://www.cdc.gov/ncidod/dhqp/pdf/ar/mdroGuideline2006.pdf (accessed Feb. 24, 2009).

11. Cohen A.L., et al.: Recommendations for metrics for multidrug-resistant organisms in healthcare settings: SHEA/HICPAC position paper. *Infect Control Hosp Epidemiol* 29, Oct. 2008. http://www.journals.uchicago.edu/doi/pdf/10.1086/591741 (accessed Feb. 24, 2009).

12. Calfee D.P., et al.: Strategies to prevent transmission of methicillin-resistant *Staphylococcus aureus* in acute care hospitals. *Infect Control Hosp Epidemiol* 29, Oct. 2008. http://www.journals.uchicago.edu/doi/full/10.1086/591061 (accessed Feb. 29, 2009).

13. Dubberke E.R., et al.: Strategies to prevent *Clostridium difficile* infections in acute care hospitals. *Infect Control Hosp Epidemiol* 29, Oct. 2008. http://www.journals.uchicago.edu/doi/full/10.1086/591065 (accessed Feb. 29, 2009).

14. Centers for Disease Control and Prevention: *Central Line–Associated Bloodstream Infection (CLABSI) Event.* www.cdc.gov/nhsn/PDFs/pscManual/4PSC_CLABScurrent.pdf (accessed May 20, 2009).

15. Marschall J., et al.: Strategies to prevent central line-associated bloodstream infections in acute care hospitals. *Infect Control Hosp Epidemiol* 29, Oct. 2008. http://www.journals.uchicago.edu/doi/full/10.1086/591059 (accessed Feb. 29, 2009).

16. Centers for Disease Control and Prevention: Guidelines for the Prevention of Intravascular Catheter-Related Infections. *MMWR Recomm Rep* 51(RR-10):1–33, Aug. 9, 2002.

17. Anderson D.J., et al.: Strategies to prevent surgical site infections in acute care hospitals. *Infect Control Hosp Epidemiol* 29, Oct. 2008. http://www.guideline.gov/summary/summary.aspx?ss=15&doc_id=13399&nbr=6810 (accessed Feb. 28, 2009).

18. Mangram A.J., et al.: CDC guideline for prevention of surgical site infection, 1999. *Infect Control Hosp Epidemiol* 20, Apr. 1999. http://www.cdc.gov/ncidod/dhqp/pdf/guidelines/SSI.pdf (accessed Feb. 28, 2009).

19. Association of PeriOperative Registered Nurses (AORN): *Perioperative Standards and Recommended Practices, 2009 Edition.* Denver: AORN, 1999.

20. Klevens R.M., et al.: Estimating health care-associated infections and deaths in U.S. hospitals, 2002. *Public Health Rep* 122:160–165, Mar.–Apr. 2007.

21. The Joint Commission: *Sentinel Event Policy and Procedures.* Jul. 2007. http://www.jointcommission.org/SentinelEvents/PolicyandProcedures (accessed Oct. 12, 2009).

22. Carrico R., Ramirez J.: A process for analysis of sentinel events due to health care–associated infection. *Am J Infect Control* 35:501–507, Oct. 2007.

Chapter 12

The Joint Commission Accreditation Process

Louise Kuhny, R.N., M.P.H., M.B.A., C.I.C.; and Barbara Moore Soule, R.N., M.P.A., C.I.C.

The Joint Commission's accreditation process moves organizations beyond survey preparation to systems improvement by focusing on how systems and processes function within a health care organization to provide safe, high-quality care, treatment, and services.

The systems and processes to survey, prevent, and control infection permeate an entire organization; a lack of attention in this area can put patient safety at risk, cause adverse outcomes, and incur increased expenses. Because it significantly impacts an organization's provision of safe, high-quality care, it is not surprising that infection prevention and control (IPC) is evaluated in multiple ways during the accreditation process. This chapter offers a brief look at the areas in which infection prevention and control is addressed. For a complete discussion of the accreditation process, see the *Comprehensive Accreditation Manual* for your program.

THE PERIODIC PERFORMANCE REVIEW

The Periodic Performance Review (PPR) process is a key component of accreditation for most health care programs. It is designed to help organizations incorporate Joint Commission standards as part of routine operations and ongoing quality improvement efforts.

In the PPR process, organizations can assess their compliance with infection prevention and control–related standards and National Patient Safety Goals, such as those discussed within this publication. For information on the complete PPR process, see your program's *Comprehensive Accreditation Manual*.

THE PRIORITY FOCUS PROCESS

The Priority Focus Process (PFP) guides the surveyor(s) in planning and conducting an organization's on-site survey. This process focuses survey activities on the organization-specific issues most relevant to safety and quality of care (referred to as *priority focus areas* [PFAs]). The PFP can be considered a process for standardizing the PFAs for review during survey.

The PFP is an open process. It uses an automated tool, which takes available data from a variety of sources—including e-Apps for accreditation, previous survey findings, complaint data, and publicly available external data—and integrates them to identify clinical/service groups (CSGs) and PFAs for an organization. (*See* Sidebar 12-1 on page 140 and Sidebar 12-2 on page 140.) The PFP converts these data into information that focuses survey activities, increases consistency in the accreditation process, customizes the accreditation process to make it specific to a particular organization, and guides tracer activities. (*See* pages 140–145 for more information on the tracer methodology.)

An organization will receive PFP information for its top PFAs and CSGs on its secure extranet site. Complex organizations surveyed under more than one accreditation program will receive program-specific PFP information and organization-level PFP information that is a summary of all programs' data and information. PFP data are updated quarterly, as changes warrant. **Note:** *Organizations will receive an updated report only if there is a change to one or more PFAs and/or CSGs in their programs since the previous PFP Report. Due to the systems* *nature of the PFAs and CSGs, it is possible that there may not be a change from one quarter to the next.*

Surveyors will use the PFP in the following ways:

- The surveyor(s) assigned to an organization will have access to that organization's PFP information via the surveyor extranet.

- The surveyor(s) will review the PFP information for the organization-specific PFAs as well as for organization-specific CSGs.

- As part of the planning process, the surveyor(s) will begin to assess and plan his or her tracer activities.

- During the on-site survey, the surveyor(s) will use the organization's active patient list to select tracer patients.

As the survey progresses, the surveyor(s) may find other priority areas that need addressing and may begin to focus less on the PFP suggested list and more on what he or she is finding.

TIP: *The PFP guides the surveyor(s) in planning and conducting an organization's on-site survey. This process focuses survey activities on the organization-specific issues most relevant to safety and quality of care.*

Sidebar 12-1: Clinical/Service Groups

Clinical/service groups (CSGs) categorize patients and/or services into distinct populations for which data can be collected. The Joint Commission created the list of CSGs based on data gathered from e-Apps from each accreditation program and on publicly available data from external sources. The list then underwent a thorough review to make sure that all categories were actually representative of populations served or services provided by the organizations surveyed by the individual accreditation programs. Joint Commission surveyors use an organization's CSGs combined with other organization-specific data to get a better understanding of the organization's systems and the patients it serves. As previously mentioned, tracer patients can be selected according to CSGs.

THE UNANNOUNCED SURVEY

The unannounced full survey is the on-site evaluation piece of the Joint Commission's accreditation process. An organization can have an unannounced survey between 18 and 39 months after its previous full unannounced survey. A survey is designed to be individualized to each organization, to be consistent, and to support the organization's efforts to improve performance. Within the unannounced survey, the

---

Sidebar 12-2: The Priority Focus Areas

Priority focus areas (PFAs) are processes, systems, or structures in a health care organization that significantly impact safety and/or the quality of care provided. The list of PFAs was developed from information gathered through Joint Commission experience, published literature, and consensus.

The PFAs are the following:
- Assessment and Care/Services (not applicable to laboratories)
- Analytic Procedures (applicable to laboratories only)
- Communication
- Credentialed Practitioners
- Equipment Use
- Infection Control
- Information Management
- Medication Management (not applicable to laboratories)
- Organizational Structure
- Orientation & Training .
- Patient Safety
- Physical Environment
- Quality Improvement Expertise/Activities
- Rights & Ethics
- Staffing

It is important to remember that the PFAs do not stand alone. They often link to each other because care systems and care processes are highly integrated and interdependent. For example, infection prevention and control intersects with many other processes and systems in a health care organization, and infection prevention and control processes may be identified for recommendations when other PFAs are being reviewed.

surveyor assesses an organization's performance and compliance with applicable standards based on the following:

- Tracing the care delivered to patients
- Verbal and written information provided to the Joint Commission
- On-site observations and interviews by Joint Commission surveyors
- Documents provided by the organization
- Specific sessions that address particular issues

Although all these methods for assessing standards compliance are important, tracer methodology is probably the most critical in getting a picture of an organization's overall performance as well as its performance in particular areas, such as infection control. The following sections take a closer look at tracer methodology.

TIP: A survey is designed to be individualized to each organization, to be consistent, and to support the organization's efforts to improve performance.

TRACER METHODOLOGY

The tracer methodology is the cornerstone of the Joint Commission on-site survey. It is a way to analyze a health care organization's system of providing care, treatment, and services using actual patients as the framework for assessing standards compliance. Within this methodology, surveyors follow the experience of care for a number of individuals (initially identified by CSGs and PFAs) through the organization's entire health care process. This allows the surveyor(s) to identify performance issues in one or more steps of the process or in the interfaces between processes.

Tracer methodology has been effective for surveyors and organizations to assess what is happening in an organization. Tracers engage the staff who provide care, treatment, and services; observe transitions and handoffs for the patients, clients, or residents; include a review of critical environmental issues; and evaluate employee knowledge and performance. Tracers that are performed well—with good interview techniques, validation of information, integrated learning, and feedback that acknowledges excellent performance and needed improvement—can be powerful tools for improving the safety and quality of care, treatment, and services provided by an organization.

There are different types of tracers during which infection prevention and control issues are addressed. Following is a brief discussion of those tracers.

TIP: Tracers engage the staff who provide care, treatment, and services; observe transitions and handoffs for the patients, clients, or residents; include a review of critical environmental issues; and evaluate employee knowledge and performance.

Individual Tracers

Individual tracers are used to "trace" the care experiences that a patient had while at the health care organization and to determine standards compliance as it relates to care delivered to the selected individual. (*See* Sidebar 12-3 for a discussion of how individuals are chosen for tracers.) During the individual tracer activity, the surveyor(s) will do the following:

- Follow the course of a type of care, treatment, or service provided to the patient by the organization
- Assess the interrelationships among disciplines and services/programs and the important functions in the care, treatment, and services provided
- Evaluate the performance of processes relevant to the

Sidebar 12-3: Selecting Individuals to Trace

When selecting patients for individual tracers, the surveyor(s) uses the following general criteria:

- Patients in top clinical/service groups (CSGs) for that organization
- Patients who cross programs (for example, long term care residents who present at a hospital or some home care patients received from a hospital in complex organizations)
- Patients related to individual-based system tracer topics, such as infection control or medication management (*see* above for more information on individual-based system tracers)
- Patients receiving complex services, such as surgery or treatment in an intensive care unit

Patients selected for initial individual tracer activity will most likely be those identified in the organization's Priority Focus Process information as listed in the CSGs.

care, treatment, and service needs of the patient, with particular focus on the integration and coordination of distinct but related processes

- Identify vulnerabilities in the care processes

Within an individual tracer, a surveyor will not only examine the individual components of a system but will also evaluate how the components of a system interact with each other. In other words, a surveyor will look at the care, treatment, and services provided by each department/unit/program and service, as well as how departments/units/programs and services work together.

The surveyor(s) may start tracing a patient where the patient is currently located. The surveyor can then move to where the patient first entered the organization's systems; an area of care provided to the patient that may be a priority for that organization; or to any areas in which the patient received care, treatment, and services. The order will vary. Along the way, the surveyor(s) will speak with the health care staff member(s) who actually provided the care to that individual tracer patient—or, if a particular staff member(s) is not available, surveyor(s) will speak with another staff member(s) who provides the same type of care.

During this tracer process, surveyors may identify infection control issues. For example, if the patient being traced has a postsurgical infection, the surveyor may begin the tracer in the preoperative care unit or the operating room (OR), the patient's room on the nursing unit, or the surgical outpatient admitting area. The areas covered during the tracer could include laboratory, radiology, physical therapy, or other relevant services. Surveyors may interview environmental services staff in the OR or on the nursing unit and interview admissions staff, emergency department (ED) staff, or staff in other areas where care is provided.

As previously mentioned, surveyors may begin a tracer where the patient first enters the care system, where the patient has not yet been but will be visiting, or where the patient will be transferred after discharge. For example, when tracing the care of an elderly individual who enters the hospital from home and is discharged to a long term care facility after treatment for pneumonia, the surveyors may trace the resident's care in the hospital and the long term care facility. If the individual is discharged to home with home health services and respiratory therapy treatments, surveyors may trace the care experience of this individual by visiting all of these settings.

Based on the findings of the surveyor(s), he or she may select similar patients to trace. The tracer methodology permits surveyors to "pull the threads" if there is a reason to believe that an issue needs further exploration.

Individual-Based System Tracers

Individual-based system tracers are interactive sessions with the surveyor(s) and organization staff that explore the performance of important patient-related functions and high-risk processes that cross the organization. Individual-based system tracers differ from individual tracers in that during individual tracers, the surveyor follows an individual through his or her course of care, evaluating all aspects of care as opposed to a "system." During the individual-based system tracer sessions, the surveyor(s) evaluates the system/process, including the integration of related processes and the coordination and communication among disciplines and departments involved with those processes.

An individual-based system tracer includes an interactive session (involving a surveyor and relevant staff members) in tracing a "system" within the organization based on information from individual tracers. Points of discussion in the interactive session include the following:

- The flow of the process across an organization, including identification and management of risk points, integration of key activities, and communication among staff/units involved in the process
- Strengths in the process and possible actions to be taken in areas needing improvement
- Issues requiring further exploration in other survey activities
- A baseline assessment of standards compliance
- Education by the surveyor, as appropriate

Infection control is one of three topics evaluated within individual-based system tracers. The infection control system tracer explores an organization's infection prevention and control processes. The goals of this session are to assess an organization's compliance with the relevant infection control standards, identify infection prevention and control issues that require further exploration, and determine actions that may be necessary to address any identified risks and improve patient safety. Discussion within the tracer may include many clinical issues as well as issues related to infection prevention and control surveillance activities and reporting processes. Prevention and control activities, including infection prevention and control training, education, housekeeping procedures, and physical facility changes, may also be addressed during this tracer.

The number of individual-based system tracers varies based on survey length. If survey length does not permit the conduct of an infection control system tracer, this area is assessed through other survey activities. On complex organization surveys (that is, organizations being surveyed under more than one accreditation program manual), a single infection control system tracer session may be scheduled. This session is intended to review infection prevention and control for all services provided by the organization.

Participants in the infection control system tracer should include individuals who are able to address infection prevention and control in all services offered by the organization.

TIP: *The infection control system tracer explores an organization's infection control processes, assesses an organization's compliance with the relevant infection control standards, identifies infection control issues that require further exploration, and determines actions that may be necessary to address any identified risks and improve patient safety.*

How the Infection Control System Tracer Works

The infection control system tracer will open with introductions and a review of the goals for the tracer, which—as previously mentioned—include the following:

- Exploration, critical thinking, and potential problem solving about the IPC program
- Identification of potential areas of concern in the IPC program, areas for improvement, and actions that could be taken

Tracer activity will then begin in a patient/resident/client care and service area (for example, inpatient unit, outpatient treatment area, day program activity room, home visit,

clinic, OR, resident, or client room) identified by the surveyor(s) and may move to other settings as appropriate and applicable to tracing infection prevention and control processes across the organization. During the tracer, the surveyor(s) will observe staff members and engage them in discussion focused on infection prevention and control practices in any setting that is visited during this system tracer activity.

The tracer activity may end in a short group meeting with individuals responsible for the organization's IPC program. During this time, the surveyor(s) will identify potential areas of concern and gain a better understanding of the infection prevention and control system for further discussion and exploration with staff knowledgeable about the organization's IPC program. During this discussion, the surveyor(s) will draw from tracer activity experience, the organization's infection prevention and control surveillance data, other infection prevention and control–related data (for example, core measures of pneumonia or surgical site infections [SSIs]), and PFP information, when available, to create scenarios for discussion with the organization. Participants in the system tracer will be asked to discuss the following aspects of the organization's IPC program as they relate to the scenarios:

- The organization's infection prevention and control risk assessment, identification of risk priorities, and infection prevention and control plan
- How the organization identifies individuals with infections
- How individuals with infections are managed within the context of the IPC program
- Current and past surveillance activity—taking place in the past 12 months
- Type of analysis being performed on infection prevention and control data, including comparisons with external or internal benchmarks
- Reporting of infection prevention and control data—frequency and audience
- Strategies for reducing infection risk through prevention and control activities (for example, staff training, environment of care procedures, organizationwide hand hygiene, food handling and preparation, techniques used for placing invasive medical devices, and the appropriate storage, cleaning,

disinfection, sterilization, and disposal of supplies and equipment)

■ Performance improvement (PI) based on surveillance data or other information

■ Interventions for licensed independent practitioners, staff, students/trainees, independent practitioners, and volunteers that include screening for exposure and immunity to infectious diseases with which they come in contact; the assessment referral; potential testing; and immunization and/or prophylaxis treatment and counseling to those who have potentially been identified with an infectious disease

■ Physical facility changes, either completed or in progress, that have an impact on infection prevention and control efforts, such as construction and renovation

■ Actions taken as a result of surveillance and the outcomes of those actions

Organizations may share infection prevention and control data during this part of the activity to illustrate their procedures and improvement efforts. Discussion may focus on patients or residents included in infection prevention and control surveillance and reporting activities or those not yet confirmed as meeting the criteria for inclusion in surveillance data. In addition to surveyor-identified scenarios, the organization is encouraged to present examples of cases that will highlight various aspects of its IPC program. Some of the scenarios the surveyors may want to discuss, as applicable to the organization, include the following:

■ Individuals seen with fever of unknown origin

■ Individuals with typical health care–associated infections (HAIs), such as SSIs, catheter-related bloodstream infections (CRBSIs), urinary tract infections (UTIs), or ventilator-associated pneumonia (VAP)

■ Individuals admitted to the organization postoperatively for possible infection

■ Individuals placed on an antibiotic in response to results from culture and sensitivities, blood levels, or other laboratory tests used for dosing, such as peak and trough levels for vancomycin

■ Individuals placed on some form of isolation or precaution because of diagnosis of infectious disease, such as varicella, pertussis, pulmonary tuberculosis (TB), meningitis, skin infections (impetigo, lice, scabies); respiratory syncytial virus; an HAI, such as

VAP or *Clostridium difficile*; or because of multidrug-resistant organism(s), such as methicillin-resistant *Staphylococcus aureus* (MRSA), vancomycin-resistant enterococci, or *Acinetobacter* species

■ Infection prevention and control practices related to emergency management, such as the unexpected influx of patients with infectious diseases

■ Individuals placed on some form of isolation or precaution because of being immunocompromised, such as those at risk for aspergillosis from construction activities

■ Employee health infection risks, such as sharps injuries or exposure to TB

■ Changes in physical facilities that have an impact on infection prevention and control

■ Individuals with known cases of active TB or other reportable diseases

At the end of the infection control system tracer, the surveyor(s) will summarize identified strengths and potential areas of concern in the IPC program and will provide education as appropriate.

Conducting a Tracer

To help prepare for the tracer methodology process and identify potential infection prevention and control issues, organizations may want to conduct mock tracers that examine infection prevention and control–related standards and requirements. Although each tracer is unique and depends on the particular circumstances of the individual being traced or the system and process being traced, organizations should keep in mind the following factors when conducting a mock tracer:

■ Use the standards and EPs as guidelines for all tracers.

■ Use tracers as an education and management tool, not an accreditation "check."

■ Ensure that the questions used in tracers follow the relevant issues that are being raised by the tracer's findings. Use prewritten questions as a helpful guide to get started.

■ Avoid concentrating on the outcome of the tracer during the tracer and just follow the issues as they arise.

■ Engage staff and management in performing tracers.

■ Conduct tracers at less-than-optimal times, such as during the evenings, on weekends, or close to holidays. This provides a better idea of the systems' and processes' strengths at vulnerable times.

- Consider using an "unannounced" approach to conducting mock tracers. Doing so provides a more realistic impression of the overall health of the organization.
- Use a tool to record findings and provide feedback to staff.
- Use findings for acknowledgement and for PI.

Individuals from the organization selected for participation in assessing infection prevention and control–related issues during the mock tracers should be able to address infection prevention and control issues related to the major departments or areas within the organization. This group may include the following individuals:

- Any individual(s) involved in the IPC program and other individuals involved in the direct provision of care, treatment, and services or support services, including physicians, nurses, pharmacists, and individuals working in the laboratory
- Staff responsible for the environment of care, employee health, emergency management, and plant facilities
- Patient safety and quality leadership

By regularly conducting tracers, organizations can get a sense of the success of infection prevention and control efforts and can identify opportunities for improvement. Incorporating data from mock tracers into a PI program can help achieve continuous standards compliance and ensure the delivery of safe, high-quality care.

SUMMARY

This chapter provides an introduction to the Joint Commission's accreditation process. By participating in activities such as the PPR, PFP, individual tracers, and individual-based system tracers, organizations can get a true sense of their infection prevention and control efforts, identify areas for improvement, realize a comprehensive IPC program, and ensure that a focus on continuous compliance and quality care is achieved.

FURTHER RESOURCES

- The Joint Commission: *Facts About the Periodic Performance Review*. Apr. 24, 2009. http://www.jointcommission.org/AboutUs/Fact_Sheets/PPR_QA.htm.
- Joint Commission Resources: Tracer methodology 101: The MRSA–related tracer. *Joint Commission: The Source*, Mar. 2009. http://www.jcrinc.com/common/Documents/OnlineExtras/MDROPG09%20Extras/The%20MRSA-Relatd%20Tracer-March%202009-The%20Source.pdf.
- The Joint Commission: *Applied Tracer Methodology: Tips and Strategies*. Oakbrook Terrace, IL: Joint Commission Resources, 2007.
- The Joint Commission: *Mock Tracer Workbook*. Oakbrook Terrace, IL: Joint Commission Resources, 2009.
- The Joint Commission: *Tracer Methodology*, 2nd ed. Oakbrook Terrace, IL: Joint Commission Resources, 2008.

Index